PROCTOLOGICAL DISEASES IN SURGICAL PRACTICE

Edited by **Pasquale Cianci**

Proctological Diseases in Surgical Practice
http://dx.doi.org/10.5772/intechopen.71454
Edited by Pasquale Cianci

Contributors

Filippo La Torre, Diego Coletta, Marcelo De Melo Andrade Coura, Renato Pietroletti, Kasaya Tantiphlachiva, Joseph Weerts, Laurine Mattart, Serge Markiewicz, Benoit Monami, Vanessa Verdin, Christian Wahlen, Adam Dziki, Radzislaw Trzcinski, Colin Peirce, Muhammad Fahad Ullah, Pasquale Cianci

First published in London, United Kingdom, 2018 by IntechOpen
IntechOpen is the global imprint of INTECHOPEN LIMITED, registered in England and Wales, registration number: 11086078, The Shard, 25th floor, 32 London Bridge Street
London, SE19SG – United Kingdom
Printed in Croatia

British Library Cataloguing-in-Publication Data
A catalogue record for this book is available from the British Library

Additional hard copies can be obtained from orders@intechopen.com

Proctological Diseases in Surgical Practice, Edited by Pasquale Cianci
p. cm.
Print ISBN 978-1-78923-634-7
Online ISBN 978-1-78923-635-4

For EU product safety concerns:
IN TECH d.o.o., Prolaz Marije Krucifikse Kozulić 3, 51000 Rijeka, Croatia,
info@intechopen.com or visit our website at intechopen.com.

Meet the editor

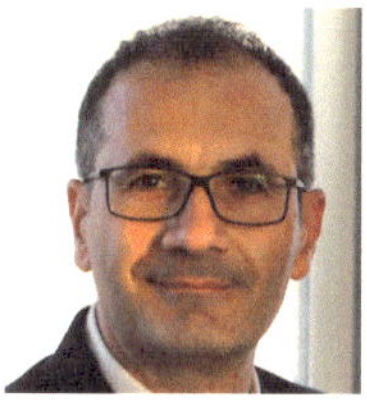

Dr. Pasquale Cianci is a general surgeon and received his PhD degree from the Department of Medical and Surgical Sciences, University of Foggia, Italy. He is a contract professor of General and Emergency Surgery, Gastroenterology, and Human Physiology at the Faculty of Medicine—Nursing Science and Physiotherapy Courses. He is a professor of Surgical Anatomy at the Specialty School in General Surgery. He is a contract professor of I Level Masters: Intestinal Stoma Care Nurse, Operating Room Nurse, and Emergency Medicine and Critical Area. He is a member of several Italian surgical societies: ACOI, SPIGC, and SIUCP. He has authored 42 scientific papers and book chapters, which are well appreciated in the scientific community. He is a reviewer of international scientific journals: WJSO, WJG, CSS, OMCR, BMJCR, and IJMPCR. He is a speaker at numerous surgical congresses. His special interests are laparoscopic surgery, endocrine surgery, and coloproctology.

Contents

Preface

Anorectal disorders are common conditions. Their prevalence in the general population is probably much higher than that seen in clinical practice as most patients do not seek medical attention. Proctology is the specialized branch of general surgery that studies anorectal diseases. Proctology was initiated late and developed slowly over the years. However, in the last 20 years, a renewed interest has begun, thanks to the contribution of many authors. This book is intended for general surgeons who are dedicated to anorectal diseases. It could also aid students undergoing specialist training. The topics covered examine uncommon aspects of these pathologies. The chapters of this book written by the authors are internationally recognized and esteemed. Each of them has inserted his personal experience in order to make the topics even more complete and interesting. In conclusion, I would like to thank all those who have helped and supported me in this ambitious, long, and demanding job, and in particular, a special thanks go to my wife Giusy and my two sons Michele and Alessandra who have always supported me.

Dr. Pasquale Cianci, MD, PhD
Department of Medical and Surgical Sciences
University of Foggia
Italy

Section 1

Introduction

Chapter 1

Introductory Chapter: A Surgical Point of View on Proctology

Pasquale Cianci

Additional information is available at the end of the chapter

http://dx.doi.org/10.5772/intechopen.79661

1. Introduction

Proctology is the specialized branch of general surgery that studies anorectal diseases. Anorectal disorders are common conditions. Their prevalence in the general population is probably much higher than that seen in clinical practice as most patients do not seek medical attention. There is no prevalence of sex, men and women of any age can be affected. The spectrum of anorectal disorders ranges from benign to potentially life-threatening (anorectal cancer). Gupta [1] divided the anorectal lesions into common, less common, and uncommon (**Table 1**). The symptoms are often not specific and difficult to evaluate; cultural and social constraints make it difficult for some patients to talk about problems in anal disorders, and doctors do not always ask patients about potential symptoms, which can delay diagnosis. In a study conducted in France, Abramovitz et al. [2] contacted 39 doctors who have joined

Common	Less common	Uncommon
Hemorrhoids	Pilonidal sinus disease	Strictures of anal canal or rectum
Anal fissures	Neoplasm	Solitary rectal ulcer
Anal fistula	Condylomas	Incontinence
Abscesses	Connective tissue masses	
Polyps	Antibioma (organized abscess)	
Rectal prolapse	Inflammatory conditions	
Anal skin tags or sentinel pile	Inflammatory bowel disorders	
Anorectal sepsis	Hypertrophied anal papillae	

Table 1. Common anorectal diseases [1].

Symptoms	Patients coming spontaneously for a proctological problem (n/%)	Proctological problem after questioning (n/%)	p-Value (Fisher's exact test)
Bleeding	8 (40.0)	41 (30.8)	0.4
Pain	12 (60.0)	35 (26.3)	0.004
Anal lump	2 (10.0)	31 (23.3)	0.2
Anal discharge	4 (20.0)	18 (13.5)	0.5
Uncontrolled anal leakage	0	22 (16.5)	0.08
Constipation	4 (20.0)	47 (35.3)	0.2
Diarrhea	1 (5.0)	11 (8.3)	1.0
Pruritus ani	8 (40.0)	26 (19.6)	0.08

Table 2. Main symptoms of anorectal diseases and their percentages without and after the questionnaire [2].

through the use of a questionnaire; the results obtained showed the main symptoms of anorectal diseases and their percentages without and after the questionnaire (**Table 2**).

2. History and proctological examination

Evaluation of anorectal disorders comprises of a careful history and physical examination before the patient can be subjected to various investigations. These disorders are commonly encountered in general surgical practice, and patients are usually in pain, often anxious and frequently embarrassed by the examination. A careful detection of anorectal and gastrointestinal symptoms (GI) and the presence of systemic disease clarify the diagnosis of most anorectal disorders. It is useful to ask standard questions to the patient about time and circumstances of onset of symptoms, duration, quality, and eventual exposure to radiation. Alterations in bowel habits should be noted: changes in color, frequency, or consistency of the stool and the presence of straining, flatus, and incontinence of solid or liquid stool. The presence of Crohn's disease, cancer, and polyps can favor the appearance of uncommon forms of anorectal problems. However, also systemic diseases such as acquired immunodeficiency syndrome, gastrointestinal malignancies, diabetes mellitus, and coagulopathy are prone to develop more serious complications of standard anorectal conditions. Patients should provide information directly to the examiner physician about sexual practices involving the anus [3]. The physical examination should take place in private, with the patient's modesty respected. The patient can then relax the external sphincter to facilitate a complete examination. The choice of position depends on the equipment available, the examiner's preference and experience, and the patient's habitus. Most frequent positions for proctologic examinations are three: lithotomic, knee-elbow position, and left lateral; the last is usually the most used in surgery (**Figure 1**) [4]. The lithotomy position allows for direct doctor-patient communication—with eye contact maintained—and patient comfort; knee-elbow position facilitates the inspection of the perianal region but it is relatively uncomfortable for the patient; the left lateral position is comfortably and readily practicable, even with very obese patients, and allows for proctologic exams

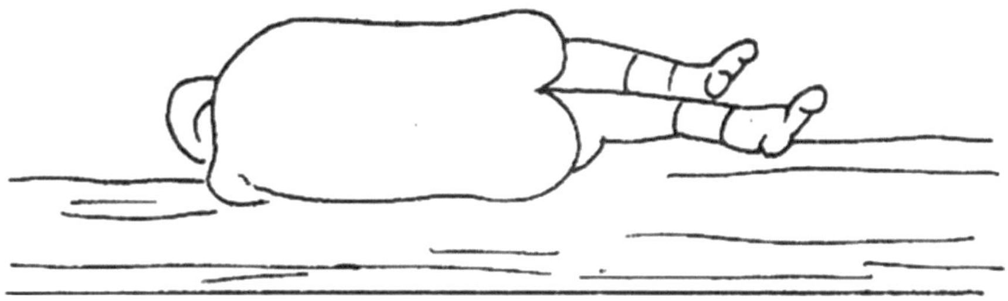

Figure 1. Left lateral position for proctologic examinations.

even on classic examination tables or on patient beds [5]. Digital rectal examination should not be missed. Through a lubricated glove, finger is placed at the anal verge and gently inserted through the anal canal into the rectum. Rectal mucosa is examined for benign or malignant lesions. It is possible to feel at least 10 cm from anal verge and perform an anal sphincter evaluation at rest and in contraction. Anoscopy and proctoscopy can help to examine of the lower part of rectum and anal canal through a proctoscope. Through this examination, we can evaluate the presence of hemorrhoids, internal opening of the fistulous tract, anal polyps, fissures, and ulceration can be identified. To date, this examination has lost interest and has been replaced by the most complete colonoscopy.

3. New perspectives

Anorectal diseases have long been considered of little interest; their treatment was considered of little prestige despite the social impact they cause to patients. Proctology was born late and developed slowly over the years. However, in the last 20 years, a renewed interest has been affirmed, thanks to the contribution of authors such as Antonio Longo who with his theory of unit prolapse and the description of innovative surgical interventions (hemorrhoidopexy, STARR, Transtar, POPS, and SIR) has been able to stimulate the interest of many surgeons in the world in regards to pathologies considered of minor importance. Today, we can affirm that important results have been achieved in the treatment of hemorrhoidal pathology, the treatment of fissures, abscesses and fistulas, obstructed defecation syndrome, rectal prolapse, pelvic floor functional disorders, and fecal incontinence. These positive results have allowed a very high percentage of healing in respect of the anatomical and/or functional integrity of the sphincter apparatus and with greater acceptance by patients. All this has been possible due to the specific professional competence acquired by proctologists, and to the more precise anatomo-clinical definition and the more accurate physiopathological interpretation of the various morbid manifestations. When necessary, a multidisciplinary approach was implemented with the integration of the skills of the proctologist, the urologist, the gynecologist, and the radiologist. Fistula-in-ano, obstructed defecation, and fecal incontinence are still major surgical challenges. The high rate of surgical failure and the need for repeat surgery are common experiences of physicians dealing with these conditions. One reason for these poor results is the lack of comprehensive knowledge about the pathophysiology of these diseases, and therefore, surgery treats the symptoms and not the causes. In the last decade, funding opportunities for benign anorectal disease research have increased vastly. The turning point was a better comprehension of anatomic damage, determined by magnetic resonance imaging and endoanal-endorectal ultrasound. The latter is becoming the paramount diagnostic instrument for use by colorectal surgeons, as it allows a clear understanding of underlying anatomic defects. Through the use of new diagnostic technologies (2D-3D endoanal ultrasonography and pelvic-perineal MRI) and morphofunctional diagnostic methods (anorectal manomentry, defecography, defeco-TC, defeco-RMN, anal electromyography, and evaluation of motor latency time pudendal nerve), a better anatomical and physiological definition was possible which allowed to better define the clinic aspects and the therapy. Generally, proctology is associated with pathologies such as hemorrhoids, fistulas, and anal fissures; in this book, we have preferred to deal with lesser known topics concerning new pre- and post-operative instrumental diagnostic techniques and of less frequent morbid conditions such as fecal incontinence and rectal prolapse with a reference also to the malignant pathology of the colon-rectum.

Author details

Pasquale Cianci

Address all correspondence to: ciancidoc1@virgilio.it

Department of Medical and Surgical Sciences, University of Foggia (Unifg), Foggia, Italy

References

[1] Gupta PJ. A review of ano-rectal disorders and their treatment. Bratislavské Lekárske Listy. 2006;**107**(8):323-331

[2] Abramowitz L, Benabderrahmane M, Pospait D, Philip J, Laouénan C. The prevalence of proctological symptoms amongst patients who see general practitioners in France. The European Journal of General Practice. 2014;**20**:301-306

[3] Gopal DV. Diseases of the rectum and anus: A clinical approach to common disorders. Clinical Cornerstone. 2002;**4**:34

[4] Shamsi Z, Anwar MA, Khan N. Rigid proctosigmoidoscopy. The Journal of the Pakistan Medical Association. 1989;**39**(7):192-194

[5] Kreuter A. Proctology—Diseases of the anal region. Journal der Deutschen Dermatologischen Gesellschaft. 2016;**14**(4):352-373

Section 2

New Developments in Endoanal and Endorectal Ultrasonography

Chapter 2

Applications of Anorectal Ultrasound in Anorectal Disorders

Kasaya Tantiphlachiva

Additional information is available at the end of the chapter

http://dx.doi.org/10.5772/intechopen.78326

Abstract

Endoanal ultrasound (EAUS) and endorectal ultrasound (ERUS) have been introduced to clinical use since the 1980s. The techniques have been used to assess various anorectal disorders and conditions, including anorectal abscess and fistula, fecal incontinence, anorectal tumor, anorectal pain and occasionally evaluation of adjacent pelvic pathology. Information acquired includes anatomical location of disease, extent of disease, involvement of anal sphincter by disease and the status of anal sphincter. This information is valuable for treatment planning, prevention of disease recurrence, prevention and/or correction of sphincter defect and follow-up evaluation. The technique is cheap, simple, well tolerated, and repeatable with acceptable accuracy. Although the interpretation is operator-dependent, technology has developed to improved image quality such as 3D-reconstruction, peroxide-enhanced technique and volume render mode. This chapter reviews the current application of anorectal ultrasound in the common anorectal disorders.

Keywords: endoanal ultrasound, endorectal ultrasound, transanal ultrasound, transrectal ultrasound, anorectal disorder

1. Introduction

Endoanorectal ultrasound (EARUS) was first described in 1956 by Wild and Reid but was not popularized due to technological limitations [1]. Law and Bartram, in 1989, had described the technique of endoanal ultrasound (EAUS) using 2D-plastic-coned probe [1, 2] and correlated the image with histological findings of the anal canal [1]. Early use of endoectal ultrasound (ERUS) is mostly by urologist to demonstrate bladder, prostate and seminal vesicle. Pahlman et al. [3] had used rectal ultrasound for preoperative staging of rectal tumor. Konishi et al. [4],

Anorectal disorders	EAUS*	ERUS**
Anorectal sepsis: abscess/fistula	✓	=
Fecal incontinence	✓	-
Anal sphincter injury	✓	-
Anorectal pain/pelvic pain	✓	✓
Anal cancer	✓	✓
Rectal cancer	-	✓
Pelvic pathology: retrorectal/gynecological/prostate	-	✓

*EAUS: endoanal ultrasound.
**ERUS: endorectal ultrasound.

Table 1. Anorectal disorder which endoanal and endorectal ultrasound can be used.

had used ERUS to assess the depth of rectal tumor invasion in order to select the patient for local excision. However, the resolution was limited by the machine frequency [4]. After sequential developments, EARUS has become an important part of the assessment for various anorectal conditions, both benign and malignant. The operator may be a radiologist, gastroenterologist or surgeon [5].

Currently, sonography for viewing anorectal region can be performed transanally, transvaginally or transperineally [6]. Here, the focus is on the transanal technique. It is well tolerated by most patients, needs minimal preparation, no radiation exposure and can be performed in the office setting [5] and in both genders. **Table 1** categorizes anorectal disorders that could be assessed by EARUS.

2. Equipment, technique and normal anatomy

Anal canal is defined functionally from the proximal aspect of the internal anal sphincter (IAS)/levator ani muscle above down to the anal verge below [7]. This area is surrounded by IAS and external anal sphincter (EAS) [7] which persistently contract. Thus, the probe is usually in close contact with the wall of the anal canal. However, in the rectum above, the water-filled balloon is used as a conduction media from the transducer to the rectal wall.

The examining position can be left lateral decubitus, lithotomy or prone jackknife position [8]. Bowel preparation or sedation is not required except in the presence of fecal impaction or severe anorectal pain, respectively. After careful digital rectal examination, the probe is lubricated and gently inserted into the anal canal. Standard orientation is that the anterior part of the patient is at 12 o'clock, posterior part at 6 o'clock, right side at 9 o'clock, and left side at 3 o'clock [8]. If it is a two-dimensional probe, the examiner should manually advance and withdraw the probe to demonstrate each anatomical level. If it is a three-dimensional probe, the examiner should hold the probe steadily in the middle of the anal canal while the image is acquired. The three planes of analysis are (1) the deeper plane: at the upper level of anal canal where the typical hyperechoic U-shaped sling of the puborectalis muscle is seen

http://dx.doi.org/10.5772/intechopen.78326

(2) the intermediate plane: at the middle level of anal canal where the hypoechoic IAS, the perineal body and the transverse perineal muscle are seen and EAS forms a complete ring (3) the superficial plane: at the lower level of the anal canal where IAS has terminated and only hyperechoic subcutaneous part of the EAS is seen [2, 9]. **Figure 1** demonstrates normal endoanal ultrasonographic views of the anal canal at each level.

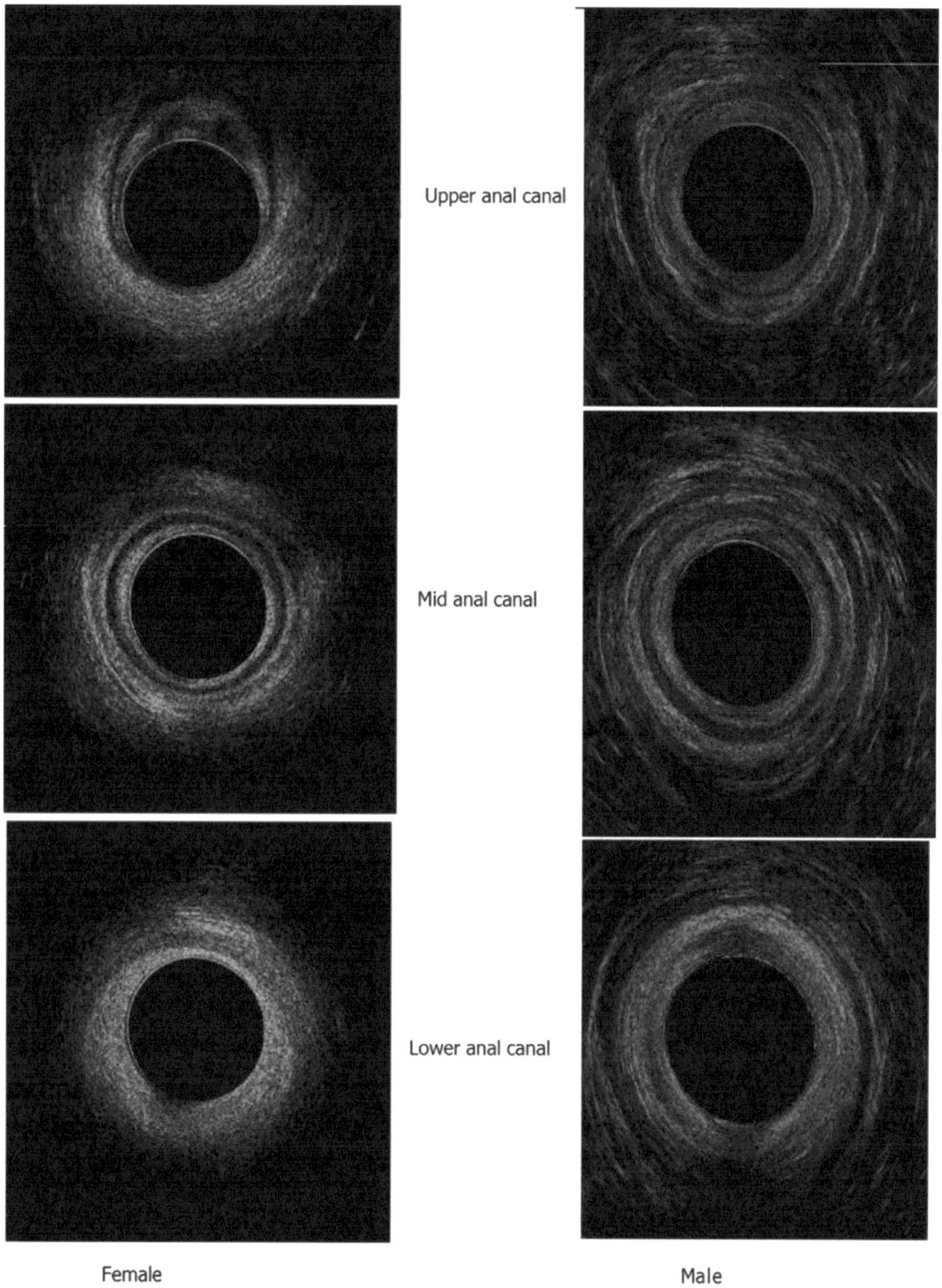

Figure 1. Normal endoanal ultrasonographic views of anal canal at three levels—left: in female and right: in male.

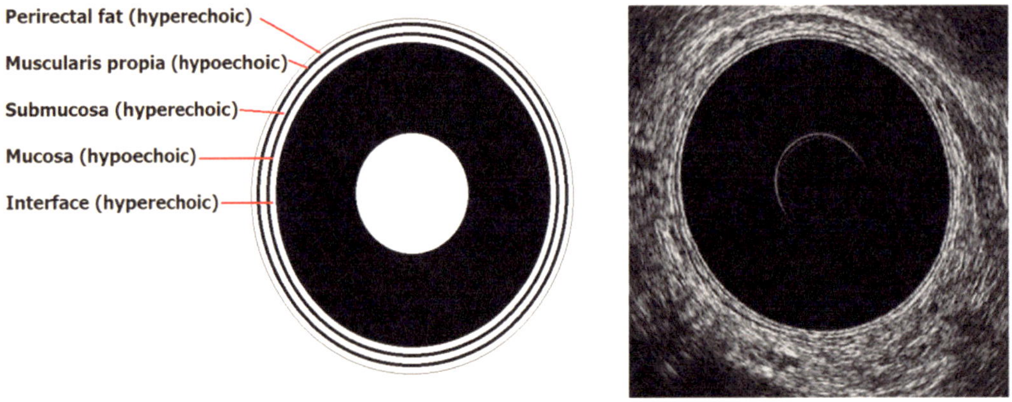

Figure 2. Endorectal ultrasonographic view of rectal wall (five layers).

Endorectal ultrasound (ERUS) views the rectal wall as alternating five hyper- and hypo-echoic layers (**Figure 2**). From the lumen outward, the innermost white (hyperechoic) layer represents the interface between the balloon and rectal mucosa. The inner dark (hypoechoic) layer represents the mucosa and muscularis mucosae. The middle white (hyperechoic) layer represents the submucosa. The outer dark (hypoechoic) layer represents the muscularis propria. The outer white (hyperechoic) layer represents the interface between the muscularis propria and perirectal fat/serosa [10, 11]. These rings should be smooth, homogenous and complete.

3. Application of endoanorectal ultrasound

3.1. Endoanal ultrasound in anorectal abscess and fistula

Most anorectal sepsis are caused by the infection of the anal gland which normally drains into anal crypts, known as cryptoglandular theory [12]. In the acute phase, the suppuration loculated in the potential space around the anus: *perianal* (or subanodermal), *intersphincteric, ischiorectal* (or ischioanal) and *supralevator abscesses* [13, 14]. In the chronic phase, the suppuration takes a course between and through anal sphincter muscles to find the exit in the perianal skin. The most commonly used classification of the anorectal fistula is Park's classification [12, 15]: *intersphincteric fistula* (primary tract courses in the intersphincteric space down to the skin), *transspincteric fistula* (primary tract traverses the EAS to enter the ischioanal fossa before exit at the skin), *suprasphincteric* (primary tract courses up within the intersphincteric plane above and over the puborectalis muscle before coursing back into ischioanal fossa downwards to the exit at the skin), *extrasphincteric fistula* (primary tract traverses levator ani to course through the ischioanal space without relation with IAS and EAS) [15]. Another additional subtype courses in the submucosa without traversing IAS or EAS is called *subcutaneous fistula* [15]. Perianal sepsis that arises from noncryptoglandular causes, such as Crohn's disease, tuberculosis, rectovaginal fistula, traumatic injury or in patients after previous anorectal surgery, may have more complex courses of the fistula and related abscess.

Preoperative imaging aims to reduce the risk of postoperative recurrences and fecal incontinence [16]. Endoanal ultrasound (EAUS) is a safe and reliable technique for the assessment of perianal sepsis [17]. With three-dimensional technology (3D-EAUS), the accuracy in identifying primary fistula type, internal opening, secondary tract and adjacent abscesses was improved from a two-dimensional view (2D-EAUS) [18]. Fistula and abscess are hypoechoic tracts or lesion within the anal wall [19]. From meta-analysis of the early studies, sensitivity and specificity for fistula detection of EAUS versus MRI were 87 versus 87% and 43 versus 69%, respectively [20]. In the identification of internal opening, sensitivity of EAUS versus MRI was 88–91% versus 19–97% and specificity of 41–100% versus 71–100% [20].

Injection of hydrogen peroxide into the external opening of the fistula has significantly improved the visualization of the fistula tract [16] as it would form into small air bubbles which show as bright hyperechoic (white) tracts [16]. The technique provided better detection of internal opening, fistula level, secondary tract and chronic fistula cavity [21, 22]. Addition of image-enhanced technology as volume rendering to the 3D-EAUS further improved the accuracy of preoperative fistula study [23, 24]. **Figure 3a** is an example of EAUS in demonstrating the horseshoe fistula using the 3D technique, hydrogen peroxide injection and volume render mode. **Figure 3b** compares the 3D-EAUS view with the rendered view of postanal space abscess.

The accuracy of EAUS in evaluation of the recurrent anorectal fistula did not significantly decrease compared to primary anorectal fistula [25]. Another useful information for planning the fistula operation, obtained during EAUS, is whether there is any anal sphincter defect(s) [25].

In Crohn-related anorectal fistula, there was no significant difference between 3D-EAUS versus MRI in detection of anorectal fistula: sensitivity, 98 versus 91%; specificity, 100 versus 100% and accuracy, 98 versus 92% [26]. While 3D-EAUS was preferable in the detection of the intersphincteric fistula, MRI was preferable in evaluation of suprasphincteric and extrasphincteric fistula [26]. EAUS technique is simple, inexpensive and well tolerated by the patient [27] and more available than MRI [28]. Thus, it is recommended as a modality for assessment of patients with occult anorectal abscess, complex anal fistula or perianal Crohn's disease [28, 29].

3.2. Endoanal ultrasound in fecal incontinence and anal sphincter injury

Fecal incontinence (FI) is a disturbing condition that greatly impacts the patient's quality of life. The anatomical causes are anal sphincter disruption or atrophy which could occur as a result of vaginal delivery, surgery, trauma or aging. EAUS is a gold standard and has an established role in defining anal sphincter anatomy and defect in the assessment of patients with FI [30–32]. Information from EAUS includes EAS/IAS/puborectalis muscle integrity, length and thickness. A comparison to the normative value may explain the possible cause(s) of incontinence [33, 34]. FI was found to be associated with anal sphincter length and thickness rather than volume [33]. IAS defect appears as a discontinuity of the hypoechoic band or localized thinning. There was a significant correlation between decreased maximal resting anal sphincter pressure and decreased IAS thickness or presence of IAS defect [35]. EAS defect appears as a discontinuity in the hyperechoic band of EAS. EAS defect or thinning was

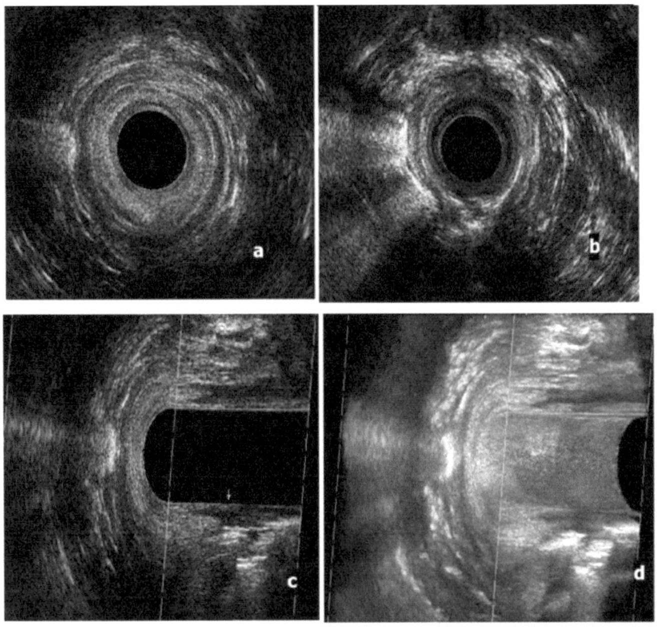

a

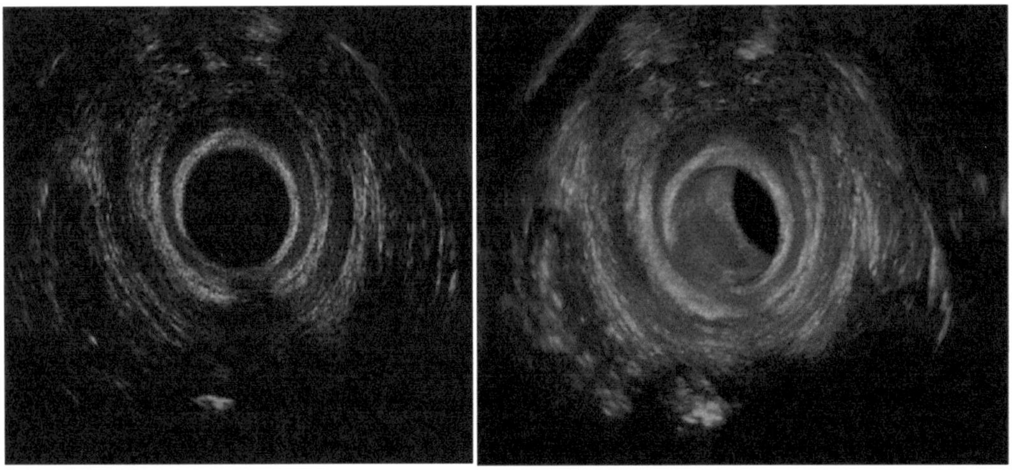

b

Figure 3. a. Endoanal ultrasound view of the right horseshoe fistula. b. 3D-EAUS view with the rendered view of postanal space abscess.

significantly correlated with maximal squeeze pressure [36]. In females, perineal body thickness measurement should be performed. The thickness of 10 mm or less is considered abnormal [37]. **Figure 4a** shows the EAUS view of anterior anal sphincter defect (most commonly found in obstetric injury) and **Figure 4b** demonstrates the perineal body measurement by

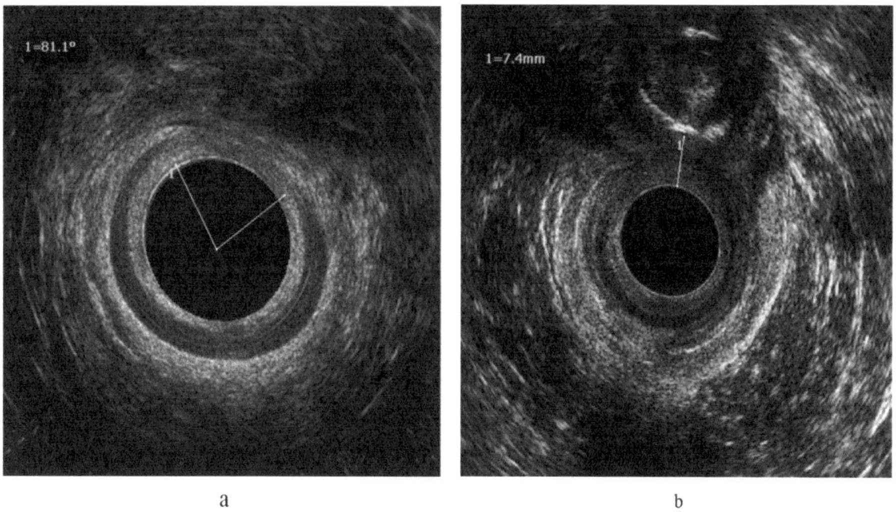

Figure 4. a. Endoanal ultrasound view of anterior anal sphincter defect; IAS defect seen as the discontinuity of the hypoechoic (dark) ring and EAS defect seen as the discontinuity of the hyperechoic (white) ring. b. Perineal body measurement; the hyperechoic shadow is the examiner's index finger that presses against the patient's posterior vaginal wall.

inserting the examiner's index finger into the patient's vagina and gently pressing on the posterior wall. Compared to MRI, 3D-EAUS can also be used to detect EAS atrophy and defects [38]. By MRI, EAS atrophy is defined as diffuse thinning of EAS or diffuse replacement of EAS by fat [38]. By EAUS, EAS atrophy is defined by the visibility of the outer interface between EAS border and subadventitial fat, reflection pattern and length [38]. The atrophic EAS could not be clearly differentiated from the subadventitial fat, has a hyperechogenic reflection, and is short [38].

In the patient who has sustained anorectal and perineal trauma, a thorough assessment of anorectal anatomy and function should be performed after the patient recovers and regains the ability to go to the toilet [39]. The preferred anorectal imaging is EAUS as the sensitivity for evaluation of anal sphincter defect is nearly 100%, better identification of IAS injury than MRI, less time-consuming and less expensive than MRI [39]. Together with the information from anorectal manometry and pudendal terminal motor latency test, a definitive treatment can be planned [30, 39].

3.3. Endoanal ultrasound in the assessment of anorectal dysfunction

3D-EAUS can be used to evaluate patients with obstructed defecation by steps of scan described by Murad-Regadas, called "echodefecography" [40]. Using this technique, anismus, anorectocele and rectal intussusception can be identified with moderate to high agreement with defecography [40]. Recent studies showed that echocardiography alone [41] or in combination with transvaginal and transperineal ultrasound is an effective and useful non-invasive test in evaluation of the patients with pelvic floor dysfunction including obstructed defecation and pelvic organ prolapse [42, 43].

3.4. Endorectal ultrasound in rectal cancer

Evaluation of rectal tumor is essential for planning the treatment. Carcinoma is seen as a hypoechoic lesion disrupting or penetrating through the rectal wall layers [11]. Villous adenoma can be classified as **uT0** lesion which does not penetrate the submucosa [11]. In situ, carcinoma (pTis) could not be differentiated from the benign adenoma using the ultrasound imaging alone [11]. A **uT1** tumor invades the submucosal layer and may be divided into uT1-slight, if only slight irregularity of the submucosa is seen, and uT1-massive, if massive irregularity of the submucosa is seen. A **uT2** tumor invades the outer hypoechoic muscular layer but with intact perirectal fat interface. A **uT3** tumor infiltrates the submucosal layer and presents as irregularity of the outer hyperechoic layer. A **uT4** tumor invades the adjacent organs such as bladder, uterus, cervix, vagina, prostate and seminal vesicles. Perirectal lymph nodes that are likely involved by the malignant cells are greater than 5 mm in size, have mixed echogenicity, irregular margins and are spherical rather than ovoid or flat [11]. **Figure 5a** demonstrates ERUS view of villous adenoma which shows no invasion of the hyperechoic middle submucosal layer. **Figure 5b** and **c** shows uT1 and uT3N1 lesions, respectively. This preoperative locoregional staging information can be used in treatment planning, whether local excision, oncologic resection or preoperative chemoradiotherapy would be appropriate.

In grossly benign rectal adenoma planning for local removal, additional ERUS may detect up to 81% of focal invasive carcinoma [44]. If the routine use of ERUS for biopsy-negative rectal adenomas is applied, the false-negative rate would be decreased from 24 to 5% and would allow better operative planning [44]. The accuracy of uT0 was 87% [45]. For other T-stages, the accuracy of preoperative uT staging is 94, 77 and 83% for T2, T3, T4, respectively [46]. From meta-analysis and a recent study [47, 48], the sensitivity and specificity for each T stages are as follows:

Sensitivity: 96, 88, 81, 96 and 95% for T0, T1, T2, T3 and T4, respectively.

Specificity: 87, 93, 96, 91 and 98% for T0, T1, T2, T3 and T4, respectively.

The concern of ERUS is that the overstaging of 18% and understaging of 13% has been reported [45]. With three-dimensional ERUS (3D-ERUS), the examiner can evaluate the arbitrary planes from any direction [49]. This improves the sensitivity, specificity and accuracy of the test [50]. For example, the sensitivity for detection of T4 is up to 100% and the specificity for T1 was 97% [50]. The total overstaging and understaging were reduced to 4.5 and 6.8%, respectively [50].

For lymph node staging, the accuracy of ERUS had been reported from 68 to 79% [45, 51]. Sensitivity and specificity were between 71 and 80% and 63 and 79%, respectively [52]. With 3D-ERUS, the accuracy improved up to 85–96% [53, 54]. Recent meta-analysis, including both 2D- and 3D-techniques, reveals sensitivity and specificity of 95 and 80%, respectively [55]. The diagnostic accuracy of ERUS for N-stage is comparable to CT and MRI [56]. Nothing is reliable in the evaluation of lymph node metastasis.

ERUS has substantial agreement with MRI and surgical pathology in predicting the radial tumor-mesorectal margin [56, 57]. From the available data, a combination of ERUS and MRI is recommended for pretreatment assessment of rectal cancer [58–60]. For postneoadjuvant chemoradiotherapy (CRT) evaluation, the accuracy to assess complete tumor response of

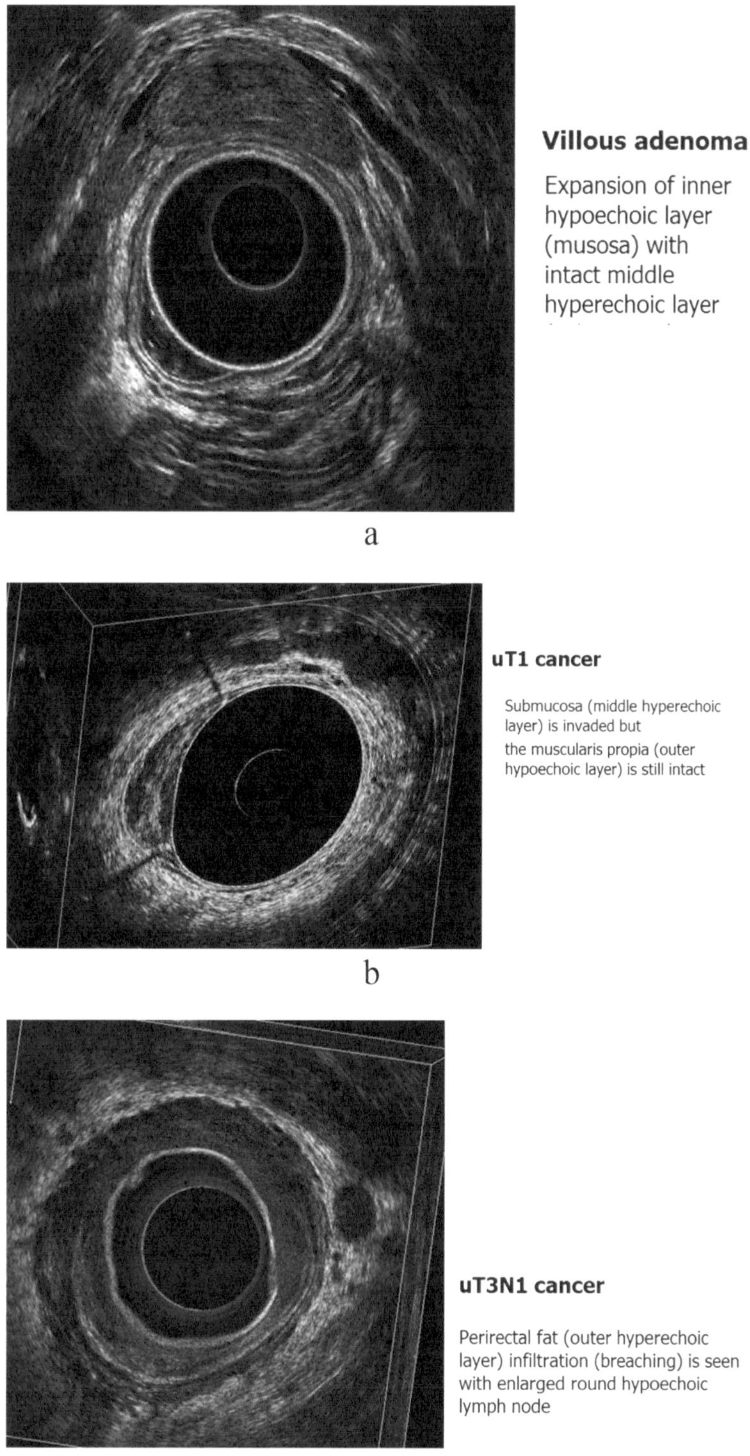

Figure 5. a. Villous adenoma, b. uT1 rectal cancer, and c. uT3N1 lesions.

ERUS, MRI and CT was 82, 75 and 83%, respectively [61]. The accuracy to detect T4 tumors with invasion to the circumferential margin was 94 and 88% for ERUS and MRI, respectively [61]. The accuracy for lymph node restaging was 72, 72 and 65% for ERUS, MRI and CT, respectively [61]. These are considered low and with no clinical relevance [61]. However, ERUS, if sequentially performed before, during and at 6–8 weeks after CRT, may predict therapeutic efficacy for locally advanced rectal cancer [62].

3.5. Endoanal-endorectal ultrasound for anal cancer

EAUS/ERUS evaluation of anal carcinoma has not been included in the major clinical guidelines [63, 64]. However, the technique is inexpensive, safe, well tolerated and repeatable for assessment of local disease [65]. EAUS staging of anal carcinoma had been proposed using the depth of invasion (**Table 2**) [65]. However, this is not correlated with the size criteria of tumor-node-metastasis (TNM) staging [66]. The exception is for T4 that the involvement of pelvic organ can be assessed. For lymph node evaluation, ERUS should be added to visualize the perirectal lymph node and any suspected lymph node should be considered as metastatic [67].

Following chemoradiotherapy, EAUS can be repeated to determine the response and used for surveillance. Although it is difficult to differentiate between post radiation change (edema, fibrosis) and tumor, tumors tend to be more hypoechogenic than scar (more mixed echogenic) [63]. It has been suggested that EAUS should not be performed within 45 days after the last radiotherapy but should be delayed until 16–20 weeks [63]. Serial examination and addition of color doppler to determine vascularity may increase the specificity in detecting local recurrence [65]. In some institutes, EAUS may be used to guide brachytherapy for anal cancer [64].

3.6. Endoanal ultrasound in anorectal pain

Endoanal ultrasound can be used in patients with chronic proctalgia to look for the possible causes, that is, chronic anorectal sepsis, IAS hypertrophy and anal sphincter defect [68, 69].

EAUS* stage	Definition
uT1	Involvement of the mucosa and submucosa without infiltration of the IAS[$]
uT2	Involvement of the IAS[$] with sparing of the EAS[$$]
uT3	Involvement of the EAS[$$]
uT4	Involvement of a pelvic organ
N0	No suspicious perirectal lymph nodes
N+	Perirectal lymph nodes suspicious for metastasis

*EAUS: endoanal ultrasound.
[$]IAS: internal anal sphincter.
[$$]EAS: external anal sphincter.

Table 2. Endoanal ultrasound staging for anal carcinoma.

Recent EAUS study found that paradoxical anal sphincter puborectalis muscle (PR) contraction during straining and increased PR thickness is more common in these patients than normal subjects [70]. This information is useful for the management plan.

3.7. Other usage

EAUS and ERUS have been used to evaluate the pathologic process around the anorectal area such as bladder lesion, ovarian tumor and retrorectal tumor [71, 72]. However, it has not been popularized and is usually used as an adjunct to other imaging modality [73].

3.8. Personal experience

Our institute, King Chulalongkorn Memorial Hospital, is a tertiary center with a colorectal surgery fellowship program. We have adopted endoanal ultrasound in our practice since 2008. By that time, the 2D-technology was used, and we had compared the data from 2D-EAUS (with selective use of peroxide enhancement) with the data from examination under anesthesia (EUA) by our most experienced surgeon, Rojanasakul A. For acute anorectal abscess, fistula-in-ano and recurrent fistula, EAUS and EUA had 67, 91 and 100% agreement in identification of internal openings, respectively (Poster presentation in the 71st colon and rectal surgery: current principles and practice 2008, Minneapolis, MN). The results are comparable to the early 2D-EAUS report [21, 74, 75]. Later, the 3D-technology was launched. We had established the normative values of the anal sphincter anatomical component [34]. The mean IAS and EAS thickness in male versus female were 1.7±0.4 versus 1.8±0.3 mm and 8.1±1.3 versus 6.9±0.9 mm, respectively [34]. The mean anal canal length in male and female was 38.6 and 34.0 mm, respectively [34]. These findings were comparable with the previous study [34, 76]. We have used intraoperative EAUS in acute anorectal abscess to guide drainage, preoperative assessment of fistula-in-ano, assessment of anal sphincter defect in patients with fecal incontinence or anal sphincter injury. ERUS has been used for assessment of rectal tumor which clinically suitable for surgery and advanced rectal cancer (preoperative staging, follow-up). Additionally, MRI is selectively used in complex cases that need further information for the multidisciplinary team and academic discussion. In our experience, EAUS and ERUS are effective, informative, inexpensive and readily available technologies for colorectal surgeons.

4. Conclusion

Endoanal-endorectal ultrasound is a useful tool for assessment of various anorectal disorders. In a static view, the anal sphincter complex can be evaluated for integrity, thickness and length as well as local staging of anorectal cancer. In a dynamic view, anorectal dysfunction and structural defects related to pelvic floor disorder can be appreciated. The technique is noninvasive, well tolerated, inexpensive and widely available. The main drawback is that the interpretation depends largely on the experience of the operator.

Acknowledgements

I would like to thank and give accreditation to Professor Dr. Arun Rojanasakul for his leadership, mentorship, inventorship and contribution to the field of colorectal surgery; Professor Chucheep Sahakitrungrueng and Assistant Professor Jirawat Pattanaarun, my teachers, for their professional teaching and introduction to anorectal ultrasound.

Conflict of interest

No conflict of interest

Author details

Kasaya Tantiphlachiva

Address all correspondence to: kasaya.tan@gmail.com

Department of Surgery, Faculty of Medicine, Chulalongkorn University, Bangkok, Thailand

References

[1] Law PJ, Bartram CI. Anal endosonography: Technique and normal anatomy. Gastrointestinal Radiology. 1989;**14**:349-353

[2] Abdool Z, Sultan AH, Tharka R. Ultrasound imaging of the anal sphincter complex: A review. The British Journal of Radiology. 2012;**85**:865-875

[3] Påhlman L, Adalsteinsson B, Glimelius B, Lindgren PG, Scheibenpflug L. Ultrasound in preoperative staging of rectal tumours. Acta Radiol Diagn (Stockh). 1984;**25**:489-494

[4] Konishi F, Muto T, Takahashi H, Itoh K, Kanazawa K, Morioka Y. Transrectal ultrasonography for the assessment of invasion of rectal carcinoma. Diseases of the Colon and Rectum. 1985;**28**:889-894

[5] Schaffzin DM, Wong WD. Surgeon-performed ultrasound: Endorectal ultrasound. Surgical Clinics of North America. 2004;**84**:1127-1149

[6] Berton F, Gola G, Wilson SR. Sonography of benign conditions of the anal canal: An update. AJR. 2007;**189**:765-773

[7] Solan P, Davis B. Anorectal anatomy and imaging techniques. Gastroenterology Clinics of North America. 2013;**42**:701-712

[8] Mihmanli I, Kantarci F, Dogra VS. Endoanorectal ultrasonography. Ultrasound Quarterly. 2011;**27**:87-104

[9] Reginelli A, Mandato Y, Cavaliere C, Pizza NL, Russo A, Cappabianca S, et al. Three-dimensional anal endosonography in depicting anal-canal anatomy. La Radiologia Medica. 2012;**117**:759-771

[10] Nasseri Y, Langenfeld SJ. Imaging for colorectal cancer. Surgical Clinics of North America. 2017;**97**:503-513

[11] Santoro GA. Preoperative staging of rectal cancer: Role of 3D endorectal ultrasonography. Acta Chirurgica Iugoslavica. 2012;**59**:57-61

[12] Parks AG, Gordon PH, Hardcastle JD. A classification of fistula-inano. The British Journal of Surgery. 1976;**63**:1-12

[13] Visscher AP, Felt-Bersma RJ. Endoanal ultrasound in perianal fistulae and abscesses. Ultrasound Quarterly. 2015;**31**:130-137

[14] Ommer A, Herold A, Berg E, Furst A, Sailer M, Schiedeck T. German S3 guideline: Anal abscess. International Journal of Colorectal Disease. 2012;**27**:831-837

[15] Sun MR, Smith MP, Kane RA. Current techniques in imaging of fistula in ano: Three-dimensional endoanal ultrasound ana magnetic resonance imaging. Seminars in Ultrasound, CT and MRI. 2008;**29**:454-471

[16] Felt-Bersma RJ. Endoanal ultrasound in perianal fistulas and abscess. Digestive and Liver Disease. 2006;**38**:537-543

[17] Brillantino A, Iacobellis F, Di Sarno G, D'Aniello F, Izzo D, Paladino F, et al. Role of tri-dimensional endoanal ultrasound (3D-EAUS) in the preoperative assessment of perianal sepsis. International Journal of Colorectal Disease. 2015;**30**:535-542

[18] Garces-Albir M, Garcia-Botello SA, Espi A, Pla-Marti V, Martin-Arevalo J, Moro-Valdezate D, et al. Three-dimensional endoanal ultrasound for diagnosis of perianal fistulas: Reliable and objective technique. World J Gastrointest Surg. 2015;**8**:513-520

[19] Kim MJ. Transrectal ultrasonography of anorectal disease: Advantages and disadvantages. Ultrasonography. 2015;**34**:19-31

[20] Siddiqui MR, Ashrafian H, Tozer P, Daulatzai N, Burling D, Hart A, et al. A diagnostic accuracy meta-analysis of endoanal ultrasound and MRI for perianal fistula assessment. Diseases of the Colon and Rectum. 2012;**55**:576-585

[21] Navarro-Luna A, Garcia-Domingo MI, Rius-Marcias J, Marco-Molina C. Ultrasound study of anal fistulas with hydrogen peroxide enhancement. Diseases of the Colon and Rectum. 2004;**47**:108-114

[22] Kim Y, Park YJ. Three-dimensional endoanal ultrasonographic assessment of an anal fistula with and without H_2O_2 enhancement. World Journal of Gastroenterology. 2009;**15**: 4810-4815

[23] Santoro GA, Fortling B. The advantages of volume rendering in three-dimensional endosonography of the anorectum. Diseases of the Colon and Rectum. 2006;**50**:359-368

[24] Sudol-Szopinska I, Kolodziejczak M, Szopinski TR. The accuracy of a postprocessing technique- volume render mode- in three-dimensional endoanal ultrasnonography of anal abscess and fistulas. Diseases of the Colon and Rectum. 2011;**54**:238-244

[25] Emile SH, Magdy A, Youssef M, Thabet W, Abdelnaby M, Omar W, et al. Utility of endoanal ultrasonography in assessment of primary and recurrent anal fistulas and for detection of associated anal sphincter defects. Journal of Gastrointestinal Surgery. 2017;**21**:1879-1887

[26] Alabiso ME, Iasiello F, Pellino G, Iacomino A, Roberto L, Pinto A, et al. 3D-EAUS and MRI in the activity of anal fistulas in Crohn's disease. Gastroenterology Research and Practice. 2016;**2016**:1895694. DOI: 10.1155/2016/1895694. Epub 2015 Dec 27

[27] Gravante G, Gordano P. The role of three-dimensional endoluminal ultrasound imaging in the evaluation of anorectal diseases: A review. Surgical Endoscopy. 2008;**22**:1570-1578

[28] Ommer A, Herold A, Berg E, Fürst A, Post S, Ruppert R, et al. German S3 guidelines: Anal abscess and fistula (second revised version). Langenbeck's Archives of Surgery. 2017;**402**:191-201

[29] Vogel JD, Johnson EK, Morris AM, Paquette IM, Saclarides TJ, Feingold DL, et al. Clinical practice guideline for the management of anorectal abscess, fistula-in-ano, and rectovaginal fistula. Diseases of the Colon and Rectum. 2016;**59**:1117-1133

[30] Albuquerque A. Endoanal ultrasonography in fecal incontinence: current and future perspectives. World Journal of Gastrointestinal Endoscopy. 2015;**7**:575-581

[31] Italian Society of Colorectal Surgery (SICCR), Pucciani F, Altomare DF, Dodi G, Falletto E, Frasson A, et al. Diagnosis and treatment of faecal incontinence: consensus statement of the Italian Society of Colorectal Surgery and the Italian Association of Hospital Gastroenterologists. Digestive and Liver Disease. 2015;**47**:628-645

[32] Paquette IM, Varma MG, Kaiser AM, Steele SR, Rafferty JF. The American Society of Colon and Rectal Surgeons' clinical practice guideline for the treatment of fecal incontinence. Diseases of the Colon and Rectum. 2015;**58**:623-636

[33] West RL, Felt-Bersma RJ, Hansen BE, Schoten WR, Kuipers EJ. Volume measurements of the anal sphincter complex in healthy controls and fecal-incontinent patients with three-dimensional reconstruction of endoanal ultrasonography images. Diseases of the Colon and Rectum. 2005;**48**:540-548

[34] Tantiphlachiva K, Sahakitrungruang C, Pattanaarun J, Rojanasakul A. Normative anatomy of the anal sphincter detected with 3D-endoanal ultrasonography. Asian Biomed. 2013;**7**:865-871

[35] Parangama C, Anu E, Sukria N. Endoanal ultrasound assessment of sphincter defects and thinning-correlation with anal manometry. Arab Journal of Gastroenterology. 2014; **15**:27-31

[36] Titi MA, Jenkins JT, Urie A, Molloy RG. Correlation between anal manometry and endosonography in female with faecal incontinence. Colorectal Disease. 2007;**10**:131-137

[37] Oberwalder M, Thaler K, Baig MK, Dinnewitzer A, Efron J, Weiss EG, et al. Anal ultrasound and endosonographic measurement of perineal body thickness, a new evaluation for fecal incontinence in females. Surgical Endoscopy. 2004;**18**(4):650

[38] Cazemier M, Terra MP, Stoker J, de Lange-de Klerk ES, Boeckxstaens GE, Mulder CJ, et al. Atrophy and defects detection of the external anal sphincter: comparison between three-dimensional anal endosonography and endoanal magnetic resonance imaging. Diseases of the Colon and Rectum 2006;**49**:20-27

[39] Jeganathan AN, Cannon JW, Bleier JI. Anal and perineal injuries. Clinics in Colon and Rectal Surgery. 2018;**31**:24-29

[40] Murad-Regadas SM, Regadas FS, Rodrigues LV, Silva FR, Soares FA, Escalante RD. A novel three-dimensional dynamic anorectal ultrasonography technique (echodefecography) to assess obstructed defecation, a comparison with defecography. Surgical Endoscopy. 2008;**22**:974-979

[41] Regadas FS, Haas EM, Abbas MA, Marcio Jorge J, Habr-Gama A, Sands D, et al. Prospective multicenter trial comparing echodefecography with defecography in the assessment of anorectal dysfunction in patients with obstructed defecation. Diseases of the Colon and Rectum. 2011;**54**:686-692

[42] Brusciano L, Limongelli P, Pescatori M, Napolitano V, Gagliardi G, Maffettone V, et al. Ultrasonographic patterns in patients with obstructed defaecation. 2007;**22**:969-977

[43] de la Portilla F, Rubio Manzanares Dorado M, Pino Dı´az V, Vazquez Monchul JM, Palacios C, Dı´az Pavo´n JM, et al. The role of tridimensional dynamic ultrasound for pelvic floor evaluation. Cirugía Española 2015;**93**:530-535

[44] Worrell S, Horvath K, Blakemore T, Flum D. Endorectal ultrasound detection of focal carcinoma within rectal adenomas. American Journal of Surgery. 2004;**187**:625-629

[45] Garcia-Aguilar J, Pollack J, Lee S-K, Hernandez de Ana E, Mellgren A, Wong WD, et al. Accuracy of endorectal ultrasonography in preoperative staging of rectal tumors. Diseases of the Colon and Rectum. 2002;**45**:10-15

[46] Xu D, Ju HX, Qian CW, Jiang F. The value of TRUS in the staging of rectal carcinoma before and after radiotherapy and comparison with the staging postoperative pathology. Clinical Radiology. 2014;**69**:481-484

[47] Puli SR, Bechtold ML, Reddy JB, Choudhary A, Antillon MR, Brugge WR. How good is endoscopic ultrasound in differentiating various T stages of rectal cancer? Meta-analysis and systematic review. Annals of Surgical Oncology. 2009;**16**:254-265

[48] Surace A, Ferrarese A, Marola S, Borello A, Cumbo J, Rivelli M, et al. Endorectal ultrasound in the diagnosis of rectal cancer: Accuracy and criticies. International Journal of Surgery. 2014;**12**(Suppl. 2):S99-S102

[49] Hunerbein M. Endorectal ultrasound in rectal cancer. Colorectal Disease. 2003;**5**:402-405

[50] Jun-hong R, Fa-jin G, Wei-de D, Xiu-jie H, Na M. Study of endorectal ultrasonography in the staging of rectal cancer. Chinese Medical Journal. 2012;**125**:3740-3743

[51] Glaser F, Schlag P, Herfarth C. Endorectal ultrasonography for the assessment of invasion of rectal tumours and lymph node involvement. The British Journal of Surgery. 1990;**77**:883-887

[52] Puli SR, Reddy JB, Bechtold ML, Choudhary A, Antillon MR, Brugge WR. Accuracy of endoscopic ultrasound to diagnose nodal invasion by rectal cancer: A meta-analysis and systematic review. Annals of Surgical Oncology. 2009;**16**:1255-1265

[53] Kim JC, Kim HC, Yu CS, Han KR, Kim JR, Lee KH, et al. Efficacy of 3-dimensional endorectal ultrasonography compared with conventional ultrasonography and computed tomography in preoperative rectal cancer staging. American Journal of Surgery. 2006;**192**:89-97

[54] Santoro GA, D'Elia A, Battistella G, Di Falco G. The use of a dedicated rectosigmoidoscope for ultrasound staging of tumours of the upper and middle third of the rectum. Colorectal Disease. 2007;**9**:61-66

[55] Zhou Y, Shao W, Lu W. Diagnostic value of endorectal ultrasonography for rectal carcinoma: A meta-analysis. Journal of Cancer Research and Therapeutics. 2014;**10**(Suppl): 319-322

[56] Phang PT, Gollub MJ, Loh BD, Nash GM, Temple LK, Paty PB, et al. Accuracy of endorectal ultrasound for measurement of the closest predicted radial mesorectal margin for rectal cancer. Diseases of the Colon and Rectum. 2012;**55**:59-64

[57] Tsai C, Hague C, Xiong W, Raval M, Karimuddin A, Brown C, et al. Evaluation of endorectal ultrasound (ERUS) and MRI for prediction of circumferential resection margin (CRM) for rectal cancer. American Journal of Surgery. 2017;**213**:936-942

[58] Gérard JP, André T, Bibeau F, Conroy T, Legoux JL, Portier G, et al. Rectal cancer: French Intergroup clinical practice guidelines for diagnosis, treatments and follow-up (SNFGE, FFCD, GERCOR, UNICANCER, SFCD, SFED, SFRO). Digestive and Liver Disease. 2017;**49**:359-367

[59] Arezzo A, Bianco F, Agresta F, Coco C, Faletti R, Krivocapic Z, et al. Practice parameters for early rectal cancer management: Italian Society of Colorectal Surgery (Societa' Italiana di Chirurgia ColoRettale; SICCR) guidelines. Techniques in Coloproctology. 2015;**19**:587-593

[60] Eberhardt SC, Carter S, Casalino DD, Merrick G, Frank SJ, Gottschalk AR, et al. ACR Appropriateness Criteria® Pretreatment Staging of Colorectal Cancer. Journal of the American College of Radiology. 2013;**10**:83-92

[61] De Jong EA, ten Berge JC, Dwarkasing RS, Rijkers AP, van Eijck CH. The accuracy of MRI, endorectal ultrasonography, and computed tomography in predicting the response of locally advanced rectal cancer after preoperative therapy: A metaanalysis. Surgery 2016; **159**:688-699

[62] Li N, Dou L, Zhang Y, Jin J Wang G, Xiao Q, et al. Use of sequential endorectal US to predict the tumor response of preoperative chemoradiotherapy in rectal cancer. Gastrointestinal Endoscopy. 2017;**85**:669-674

[63] Martellucci J. Endoanal ultrasound for anal cancer follow up. International Journal of Colorectal Disease. 2011;**26**:679-680

[64] Granata V, Fusco R, Reginelli A, Roberto L, Granata F, Rega D, et al. Radiological assessment of anal cancer: An overview and update. Infectious Agents and Cancer. 2016;**11**:52. eCollection 2016

[65] Parikh J, Shaw A, Grant LA, Schizas AM, Datta V, Williams AB, et al. Anal carcinomas: the role of endoanal ultrasound and magnetic resonance imaging in staging, response evaluation and follow-up. European Radiology. 2011;**21**:776-785

[66] NCCN Clinical Practice Guidelines in Oncology on Anal Carcinoma, Version 2.2017. Available from: http://www.nccn.org

[67] Jacopo M. Endoanal ultrasound for anal cancer staging. International Journal of Colorectal Disease. 2011;**26**:385-386

[68] Beer-Gabel M, Carter D, Venturero M, Zmora O, Zbar AP. Ultrasonographic assessment of patients referred with chronic anal pain to tertiary referral centre. Techniques in Coloproctology. 2010;**14**:107-112

[69] Garcia-Montes MJ, Arguelles-Arias F, Jimenez-Contreras S, Sanchez-Gey S, Pellicer-Bautista F, Herrerias-Gutierrez JM. Should anorectal ultrasonography be included as a diagnostic tool for chronic anal pain? Revista Española de Enfermedades Digestivas. 2010;**102**:7-14

[70] Xue YH, Ding SQ, Ding YJ, Pan LQ. Role of three-dimensional endoanal ultrasound in assessing the anal sphincter morphology of female patients with chronic proctalgia. World Journal of Gastroenterology. 2017;**23**:3900-3906

[71] Schaarschmidt K, Willital GH. Intraanal ultrasound: A new air in the diagnosis of pelvic process and their relation to the sphincter complex. Journal of Pediatric Surgery. 1992; **27**:604-608

[72] Hutton KA, Benson EA. Case report: Tailgut cyst-assessment with transrectal ultrasound. Clinical Radiology. 1992;**45**:288-289

[73] Zoller S, Joos A, Dinter D, Back W, Horisberger K, Post S, et al. Retrorectal tumors: Excision by transanal endoscopic microsurgery. Revista Española de Enfermedades Digestivas. 2007;**99**:547-530

[74] Cataldo PA, Senagore A, Luchtefeld MA. Intrarectal ultrasound in the evaluation of perirectal abscesses. Diseases of the Colon and Rectum. 1993;**36**:554-558

[75] Moscowitz I, Baig MK, Nogueras JJ, Ovalioglu E, Weiss EG, Singh JJ, et al. Accuracy of hydrogen peroxide enhanced endoanal ultrasonography in assessment of the internal opening of an anal fistula complex. Techniques in Coloproctology. 2003;**7**:133-137

[76] Knowles AM, Knowles CH, Scott SM, Lunniss PJ. Effects of age and gender on three-dimensional endoanal ultrasonography measurements: Development of normal ranges. Techniques in Coloproctology. 2008;**12**:323-329

Chapter 3

The Role of Three-Dimensional Endoanal Ultrasound in Preoperative Evaluation of Anorectal Diseases

Marcelo de Melo Andrade Coura

Additional information is available at the end of the chapter

http://dx.doi.org/10.5772/intechopen.76620

Abstract

Three-dimensional endoanal ultrasound (3D EAUS) has increased its application in coloproctology, both in pre- or in post-operative settings, since it provides more detailed information about anorectal anatomy and function. Perianal fistula complex, internal opening location and fistula tract relation with anal canal muscles are easily viewed on 3D EAUS. Moreover, hemorrhoidectomy, sphincterotomy and transanal rectal excisions hold potential in damaging anal sphincters and should be taken into account by the surgeon. Likewise, 3D EAUS has also a significant role in staging locoregional anal and rectal tumors with comparable accuracy to pelvic magnetic resonance imaging (MRI), particularly in regard to T staging in early lesions and tumor response after neoadjuvant therapy. Finally, patients with pelvic floor dysfunction or pelvic organ prolapse (POP) may benefit from 3D EAUS dynamic evaluation in order to rule out an occult sphincter defect or to unveil unsuspected anatomical multi-compartment dysfunction. Therefore, this review will address the current role of 3D EAUS as a valuable tool in modern colorectal surgical practice, highlighting its application in evaluating benign anorectal diseases, anal canal and rectal tumors and evacuation disorders, namely echodefecography.

Keywords: three-dimensional endoanal ultrasound, anorectal surgery, preoperative evaluation, anal physiology, rectal tumors

1. Introduction

Endoanal ultrasound was described for the first time almost 30 years ago [1]. Since then, we have witnessed its evolution and application in modern colorectal practice. There are now high-frequency probes (16 MHz) with excellent spatial resolution and automatic image acquisition, which, coupled with the development of recent software, are capable of generating high-quality two- or three-dimensional images.

3D images are generated by the coordinate movement of two crystals inside the transducer, creating automatic sequences of bi-dimensional captures without moving the probe [2]. The time spent is no longer than 55 s and the superposition of images creates a cube that enables the examiner to evaluate real time and as many as necessary, all details of anatomy in multiple planes.

The exam is performed with the patient in lateral decubitus, usually with no sedation. A previous rectal enema 2 h before the exam's scheduled time is recommended. The probe is inserted up to 6–7 or 15 cm depending on whether an anal scanning or a rectal scanning has to be undertaken.

External anal sphincter (EAS), a striated hyperechoic muscle, has very low water content while internal anal sphincter (IAS), a smooth hypoechoic muscle, has high water content. Due to these different tissue/echogenic proprieties, anorectal muscles are clearly viewed on endoanal ultrasound (**Figure 1**).

Regadas et al. have described the modern anatomy of anal canal on 3D EAUS in both genders. They pointed out anatomic misconcepts related to the sphincter disposition in the anal canal, that have been clarified when viewed in sagittal plane, and the same authors have further expanded these concepts to nulliparous and multiparous women [3, 4].

In sagittal plane, it is possible to measure the longitudinal length of anal canal, EAS, IAS and puborectalis muscle. In women, mainly who had vaginal deliveries, there is an anterior area devoid of muscle located in superior anal canal, prone to developing anorectocele. On the contrary, men have the same area covered anteriorly by the prostate, which prevents anorectal anterior wall from herniation (**Figure 2**).

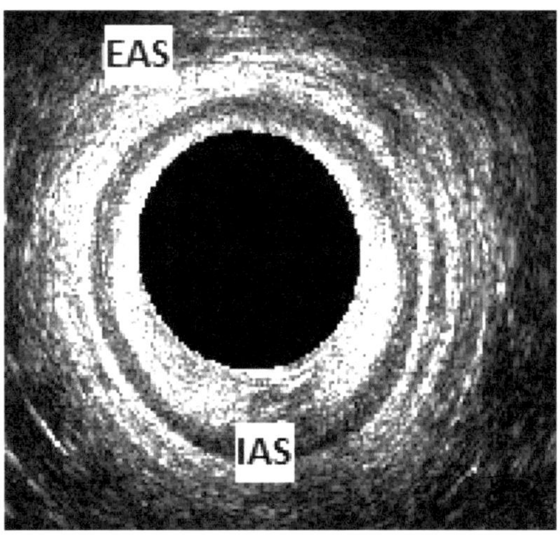

Figure 1. Detail in axial view of hyperechoic external anal sphincter (EAS) and hypoechoic internal anal sphincter (IAS). Note that they appear as two concentric rings with different echogenicity.

Murad-Regadas et al. have suggested dividing the canal anal into three regions: superior anal canal that comprises the puborectalis muscle longitudinal extension; middle anal canal that comprises the longitudinal extension of the overlapping of EAS and IAS and the inferior anal canal that comprises only of the extension of EAS subcutaneous part.

A 3D EAUS scanning of rectal layers is a more challenging exam where the examiner does need some experience in undertaking a proper capture. It is recommended that at least 30 exams should be performed in order to obtain proficiency in rectal exams [5].

A rectal scan always requires wall distention by using a balloon attached to the probe and frequently involves many insertions and lumen cleansing during the exam, in order to minimize artifacts' interference. Moreover, the probe must remain in a perpendicular axis related to the rectal lumen, throughout the image acquisition. As in anal scan, the five rectal layers are viewed on 3D EAUS as alternate layers with different echogenic properties, as depicted in **Figure 3**.

Due to these abovementioned properties and high spatial resolution, 3D EAUS has been used in modern colorectal practice to assess benign or malignant anorectal diseases both in pre- and post-operative settings. In recent years, the dynamic scan, namely echodefecography, has increased its role in routine work-up of patients with pelvic floor dysfunction, outperforming MRI defecography and conventional defecography, with better tolerance and not needing radiation.

We have been performing all 3D EAUS modalities over the last 10 years on a routine basis. The main indications still are anorectal fistula, fecal incontinence and preoperative local staging for rectal cancer. However, as the exam has evolved, the indications have evolved as well. The recent addition of transvaginal scan to ecodefecography has increased the 3D EAUS role in anorectal physiology, allowing a comprehensive evaluation of multi-compartment pelvic floor prolapse. **Table 1** shows the most common indications to 3D EAUS we have performed in over a thousand patients.

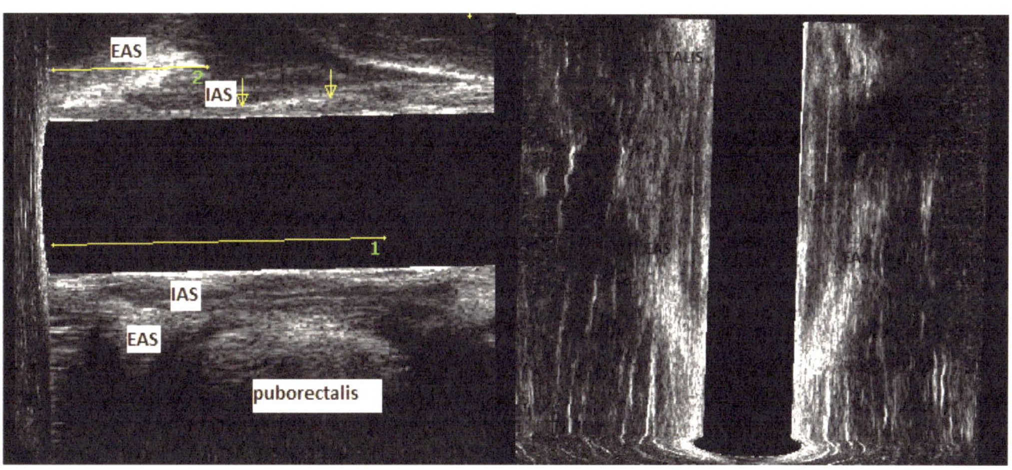

Figure 2. Multiple views of normal female anal canal. A. Sagittal view of anterior and posterior aspects of external anal sphincter (EAS), internal anal sphincter (IAS) and puborectalis muscle. B. Coronal view of right and left aspects of EAS, IAS and puborectalis muscle. Note the anterior area devoid of sphincter (arrows).

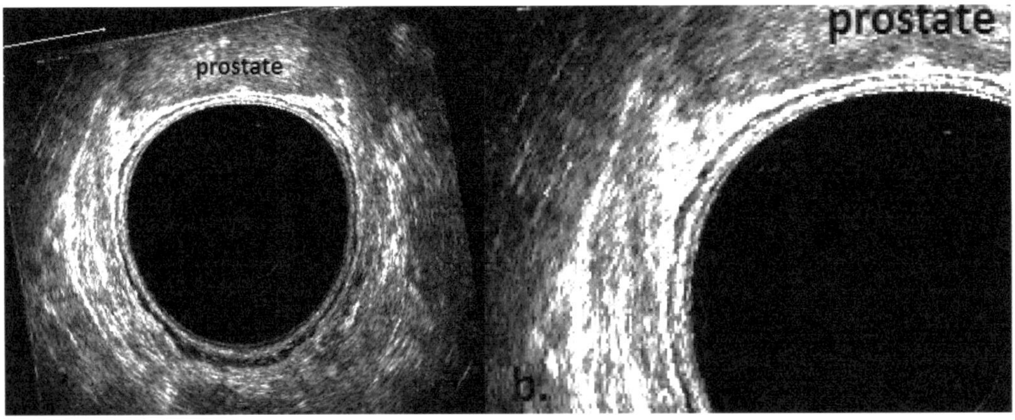

Figure 3. (a) Normal disposition of rectal layers after full balloon distension. (b) Detail of the rectal wall disposed as alternated hyper- and hypoechoic layers: mucous membrane (inner white), muscularis mucosa (next dark), submucosa (next white), muscularis propria (outer dark) and perirectal fat.

Indications	Cases (%)
Benign anorectal diseases	421 (37.75%)
Anorectal abscess	18
Perianal fistula	350
Preoperative anorectal surgery	22
Postoperative fistulotomy/sphincterotomy or sphincteroplasty	31
Malignant anorectal diseases	207 (18.56%)
Rectal tumor preoperative	143
Post neoadjuvant Rdt/Chem	52
Anal canal tumor	12
Fecal incontinence	187 (16.77%)
Obstructed defecation	212 (19%)
Pelvic organ prolapse(POP)- preoperative/ postoperative	45 (4.12%)
Other	43 (3.8%)

Rdt, radiotherapy; Chem, chemotherapy.

Table 1. 3D EAUS indications in author's personal cases.

With the basic initials concepts in mind, this review will outline the multiple applications of 3D EAUS in coloproctology, focusing as pre-operative and post-operative settings. Its role in evaluating surgical cases of benign anorectal diseases, malignant anorectal diseases and finally echodefecography, the dynamic technique assessment used in pelvic floor functional diseases, is discussed.

2. 3D EAUS in benign anorectal diseases

2.1. Perianal sepsis

Perianal sepsis refers both to anorectal abscesses (acute phase) and to anorectal fistulas (chronic phase), as different forms of the same disease [6].

Anorectal abscesses are easy to diagnose with self-evident signs and symptoms presented by patients, which prompt urgent treatment, usually by surgical drainage. However, some patients may present with fever, pelvic pain or anorectal discomfort, without overt signs in the perianal region. Due to local pain, digital rectal examination is not feasible or when possible, it is performed under difficult conditions, not capable of ruling out a deep occult pelvirectal abscess.

In this situation, 3D EAUS is a suitable imaging technique that shows location, in relation to the sphincter muscles/rectal wall, extension of cavity and sometimes the internal opening what helps guide the surgeon to the best treatment approach [7]. Usually, the exam is performed under minimal sedation with duration no longer than 1–2 min. A typical ischiorectal abscess image is easily seen and appears as a heterogeneous hypoechoic image due to some debris inside the cavity (**Figure 4**).

Irrespective of spontaneous or surgical drainage, over half of abscesses become chronic inflammatory anorectal fistula tracts [6]. 3D EAUS has played a pivotal role in evaluating anorectal fistulas tracts in the pre-operative routine work-up [7].

When the external opening is patent, it is possible to inject through this opening, first under normal pressure and then at high pressure, 0.1–0.5 ml of H_2O_2 whose bubbles will increase the fistula tract's echogenicity, showing clearly its relation to anorectal muscles, the location of internal opening (IO), accessories tracts and occult cavities [7, 8] (**Figure 5**).

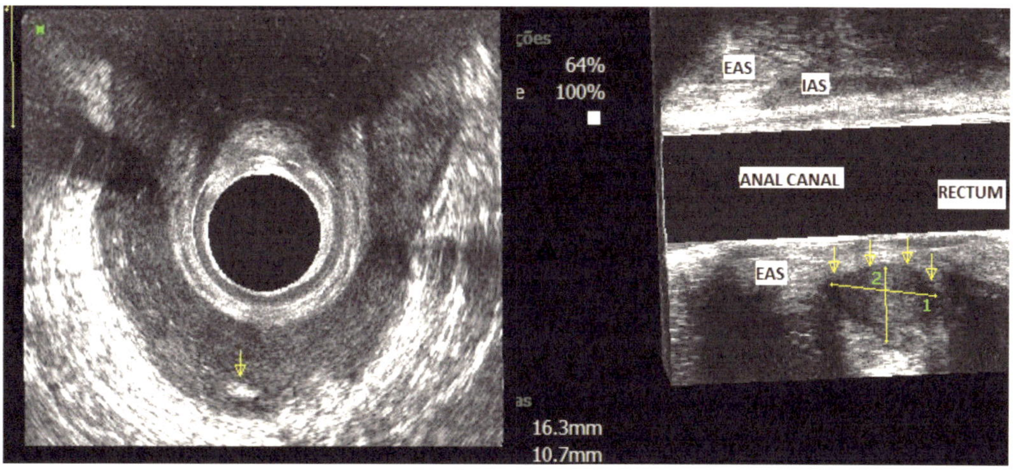

Figure 4. Left. Voluminous horseshoe ischiorectal abscess in axial view. Arrow: detail of debris seen inside the cavity. Right. Aspect in sagittal view depicting precise cavity measurements and location related to anal canal and rectum (arrows).

3D EAUS is able to drive more accurate surgical decisions by revealing accessory tracts or defining the exact location of IO not detected intraoperatively. Defining the internal opening location is not an easy task and many recurrences occur once IO or accessory tracts are overlooked during the surgical procedure [6].

Toyonaga et al. analyze a prospective series of 400 patients and were able to demonstrate that 3D EAUS was superior to intraoperative findings in identifying fistula tract (88.8 vs. 85.0%, $p = 0.0287$) and on localizing IO (85.5 vs. 69.1%, $p < 0.0001$) with lesser recurrence in cases evaluated pre-operatively with ultrasound [9].

With one acquisition, 3D EAUS allows real-time, multiple views of the fistula complex revealing precisely its relation to sphincter muscles, an invaluable information in complex fistulas, namely supra-sphincteric or extra-sphincteric fistulas.

These tracts involve sometimes the whole-sphincter longitudinal extension precluding a lay open technique, when incontinence is to be avoided. Options such as endorectal advancement flaps, cutting seton, fibrin glue or ligation of intersphincteric fistula tact (LIFT) should be considered, although they are all defined pre-operatively [10]. 3D EAUS allows surgeons not just to locate IO before operation but also to measure the exact distance from anal verge and determine how much muscle is involved by the main tract, therefore, defining which is the best surgical option (**Figure 6**).

In these complex cases, it is necessary to acquire images on the rectal mode in order to diagnose IO sometimes located on the rectal wall. These cases must be suspected when external openings are distant from anal verge (>3 cm) or when no palpable tract is identified in the physical exam.

We believe almost every patient with a diagnosis of perianal fistula should have their fistula tract evaluated by imaging. Nonetheless, we recommend that women with external opening located in anterior perineum, fistula with multiple external openings, recurrent fistulas and those from Crohn's disease must have obligatory imaging examination in order to avoid incontinence or fistula recurrence.

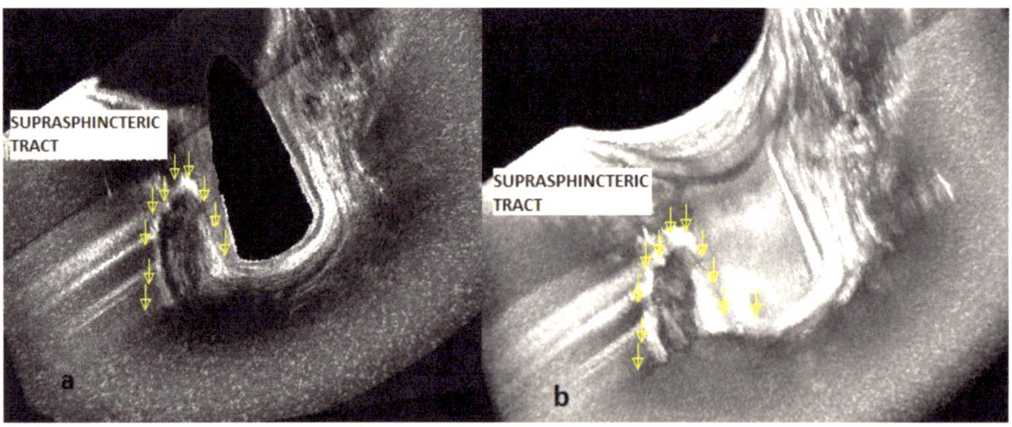

Figure 5. (a) Multiple axial and coronal views. Suprasphincteric fistula in real time 3D visualization (arrows). (b) Volume rendered mode revealing main tract orientation related to anorectal junction.

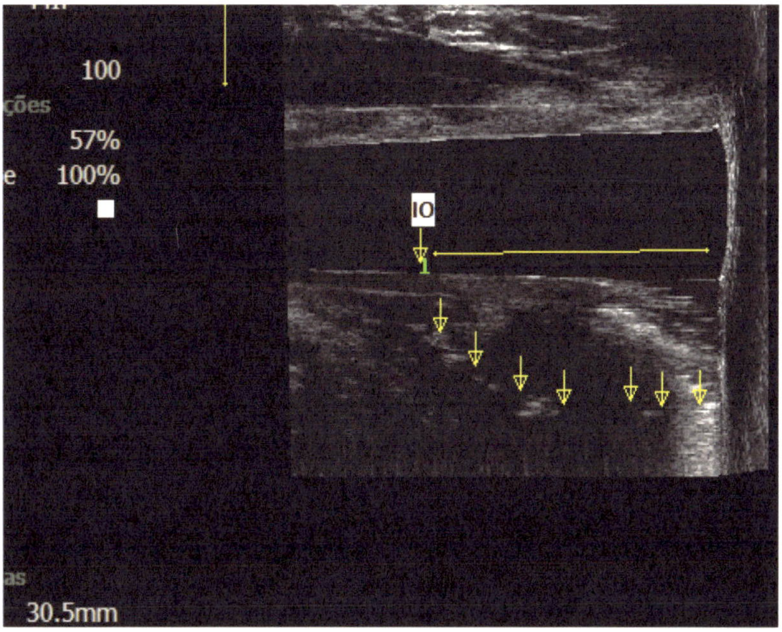

Figure 6. Sagittal view. Posterior transsphincteric fistula tract (arrows) enhanced by injection of H_20_2 through the external opening. Internal opening is located mid-posteriorly, 3 cm from the anal margin.

3D EAUS findings are heavily dependent on examiner expertise. Nevertheless, literature has supported enhanced 3D EAUS with high frequency probes, as an indisputable tool in evaluating pre-operatively patients with perianal fistulas when compared to pelvic MRI. Recent meta-analysis has shown that 3D EAUS with H_2O_2 enhancement is comparable to pelvic MRI in accuracy for both simple and complex fistulas, mostly for transsphincteric tracts, IO location and accessories tracts [11].

When reporting a typical exam for perianal fistula it is necessary to identify at least three landmarks: location of internal openings that might be located in the rectal wall, the position of main tract and relation to sphincter complex measuring how much sphincter is involved by the main tract and when present, accessory tracts. The main tract identified on ultrasound is classified by using the same types as described by Parks et al. [12].

Lastly, it is worth noting that 3D EAUS has as well a significant role in diagnosing perianal fistula recurrences. Previous surgery, scars and inflammatory process may hinder an adequate exam, influencing ultrasound results. Nonetheless, 3D EAUS is capable of diagnosing accessory tracts or IO not identified intraoperatively or even undrained abscesses as depicted in **Figure 7**.

2.2. Hemorrhoidectomy, sphincterotomy and sphincteroplasty

Many anorectal surgical procedures like hemorrhoidectomy, transanal rectal endoscopic operations or sphincterotomy hold potential in disrupting the integrity of sphincter muscles [13, 14]. 3D EAUS has been used as an adjunctive tool in evaluating such cases pre- and post-operatively.

Hemorrhoidopexy, by using transanal staplers, involves stapling mucosa and submucosa layers in anorectal junction, where lies the hemorrhoidal complex. In this technique, internal anal sphincter and more rarely external anal sphincter are prone to injury during the stapler firing—what may cause long-term rectal pain or fecal incontinence [15].

In this regard, 3D EAUS is suitable to disclosing sphincter defects pre-operatively and, more importantly, identifies some muscle involvement after hemorrhoidopexy.

Likewise, transanal rectal endoscopic operations require introducing a large proctoscope for better assessment and visualization of rectal lumen in order to properly resect rectal tumors, what may stretch or even disrupt the circular sphincter integrity. Therefore, 3D EAUS as indicated for evaluating the rectal tumors in itself should pay close attention to sphincter integrity as well.

Lateral sphincterotomy was devised to intentionally divide the distal part of IAS in patients with chronic anal fissure not responsive to clinical treatment. In this situation, 3D EAUS coupled to anorectal manometry are obligatory pre-operative exams in order to assure surgeons about muscle integrity and even post-operatively to check the extension of the sphincter section (**Figure 8**).

Once all the situations above cited carry just a theoretical risk in sphincter damage, it is arguable whether every patient in a pre-operative setting should have a complete anorectal evaluation related to function or anatomy.

Nonetheless, we would like to stress that some patients are prone to develop symptoms of anal or fecal incontinence after anorectal operations, mainly older women with asymptomatic sphincter defects [14].

After vaginal delivery it is believed that over one-third of women may have unsuspected clinical obstetric anal sphincter injuries (OASIS), only detected by endoanal ultrasound. The impact on anorectal function and fecal continence in the long term is long term [16].

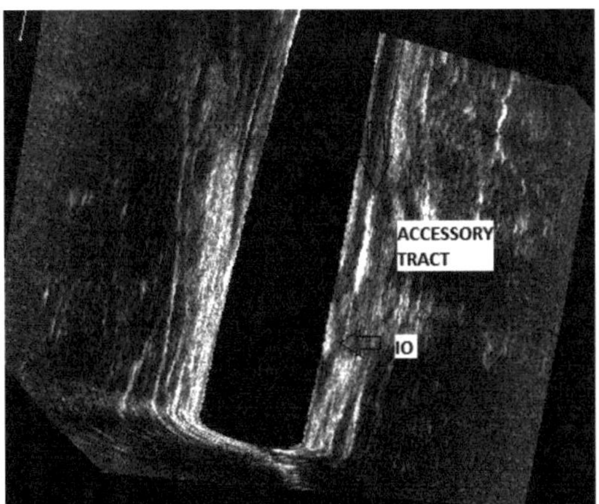

Figure 7. Recurrent fistula, 3 months after fistulotomy. Note the ascending accessory tract (upper arrow) in the intersphincteric plane. Internal orifice (IO) patent in middle anal canal.

http://dx.doi.org/10.5772/intechopen.76620

Nonetheless, a superimposed surgical procedure could, in theory, initiate or even worsen incontinence in asymptomatic or mildly symptomatic cases, respectively.

In this context, we believe it is recommended that surgeons are beforehand aware about this potential risk and make sure that anal sphincters' morphology and function are intact or even not severely damaged, by a comprehensive history, physical examination and image techniques, even though no clear-cut association between sphincter lesions and incontinence has been proven so far.

Therefore, patients who had had previous perianal operations or present abnormal anorectal manometry findings, women >60 years old specially with a history of vaginal delivery, those elected for sphincterotomy or fistulotomy and those with incontinence symptoms should have their anal sphincter and pelvic floor muscles anatomy evaluated in the pre-operative period.

Conversely, 3D EAUS should be an integral part of a routine work-up in incontinence cases, as it could add valuable information to anorectal manometry findings. For instance, patients with an identifiable defect on 3D EAUS are possible candidates to sphincteroplasty procedures depending on how severe the sphincter defect is, while cases with intact sphincters are definitely not candidates to surgical treatment [3].

Moreover, in cases where sphincteroplasty is indicated, 3D EAUS is the golden standard in identifying anal sphincter defects. It allows measuring the angle between health muscle bundles and the longitudinal extension of the defect. These findings help surgeons in better planning of the surgical procedure, taking into consideration muscles bundles quality, angle of separation and tension of overlapping. In the post-operative setting, 3D EAUS may confirm the adequacy of a surgical procedure by showing the final aspect of EAS overlapping (**Figure 9**).

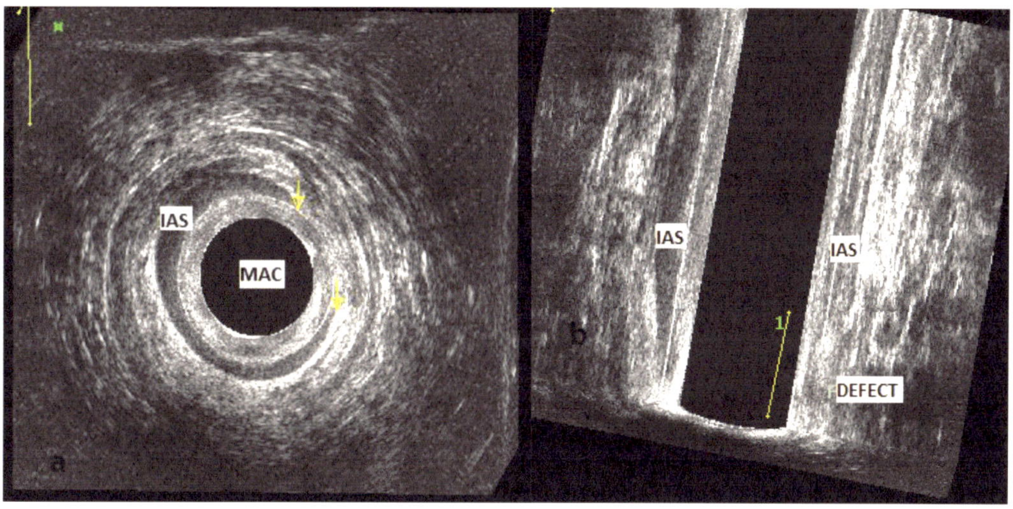

Figure 8. (a) Axial view. Lower defect of internal anal sphincter (IAS) after left lateral sphincterotomy (arrows). (b) Coronal view. Longitudinal extension of the defect.

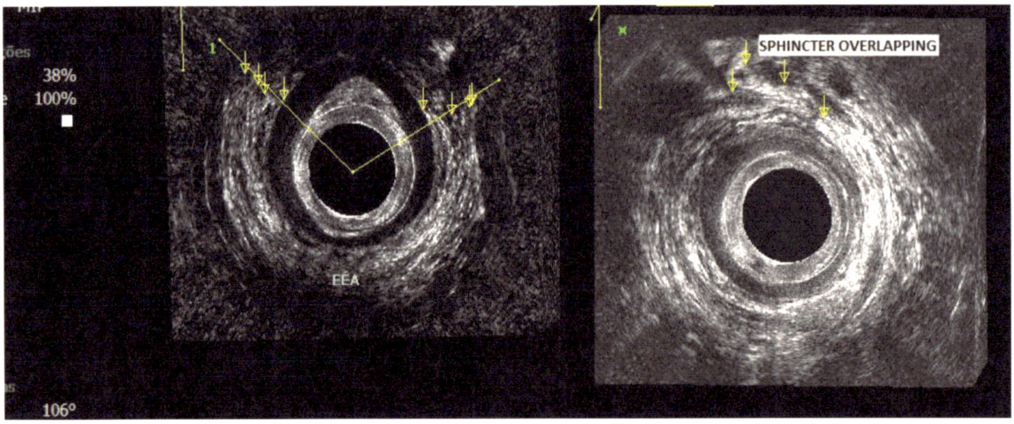

Figure 9. Complete anterior defect of external anal sphincter (EAS) after childbirth. Left: angle of muscle disruption measured by the confluence of two lines drawn from the irregular borders of EAS (arrows) to the center of the anal canal. Right: aspect 1 month after sphincteroplasty.

3. 3D EAUS in malignant anorectal diseases

3.1. Rectal cancer

Colorectal cancer is the third most common tumor in mortality worldwide and rectal cancer is responsible for over one-third of all colorectal cancer cases [17]. Recently, the widespread use of colonoscopy in campaigns for colorectal cancer screening has increased the number of cases diagnosed as early rectal lesions, hence, amenable to local excision.

On the other hand, patients with more advanced lesions frequently present symptoms as anal bleeding associated with tenesmus, rectal pain or change in bowel habits. Digital rectal examination, colonoscopy and imaging exams are necessary to accurately assess the disease and define proper treatment strategy.

Regarding local extension, both early and advanced lesions are better evaluated by 3D EAUS, MRI or a combination of both [18–20].

The aim of locoregional staging is to sort out cases to upfront surgical treatment from cases selected for neoadjuvant radio and chemotherapy, followed by re-staging and posterior definitive rectal excision [21]. In more favorable cases, rectal tumors may show a complete clinical response after neoadjuvant step. Such cases must be followed closely with serial digital rectal examination, proctoscopy and endoanal ultrasound or MRI in order to identify endoluminal, parietal or mesorectal nodal recurrence [22].

In all these situations, 3D EAUS is an important tool in rectal tumor management with accuracy comparable to MRI [5, 18, 20, 23].

Hildebrandt and Feifel have proposed a step-wise form to stage loco-regional rectal cancer based on endoanal ultrasound findings, by dividing rectal walls into five layers. These five layers show different echogenic properties, which enable accurate T evaluation, notably for early lesions T1-2 [24]. According to this classification, lesions that present thickening of muscularis mucosa with no breach in submucosa are classified as Tis tumors. In its turn, lesions with the disruption of the submucosal layer with no thickening of muscular propria are classified as T1 tumors, as seen in **Figure 10**.

Lymph nodes present in perirectal fat are easily observed on 3D EAUS. They must be evaluated up to the retrosigmoid transition, regardless of tumor location in the rectum, in order to not miss any suspect node. Lymph nodes are likely to be metastatic when they are hypoechoic, are >10 mm and show a round form and irregular borders, suggesting lymph node tissue substitution for tumor tissues [5, 26].

3D EAUS allows node differentiation from blood vessels, once blood vessels have a branch-like configuration in sagittal planes while lymph nodes are round or oval in shape, both in axial and in sagittal planes (**Figure 11**).

Acquisition in rectal scanning mode is more challenging than in anal mode, and it requires from the examiner more experience in performing the captures [5]. Typically, it demands multiple insertions in order to clean up rectal lumen to minimize artifact interference. Likewise,

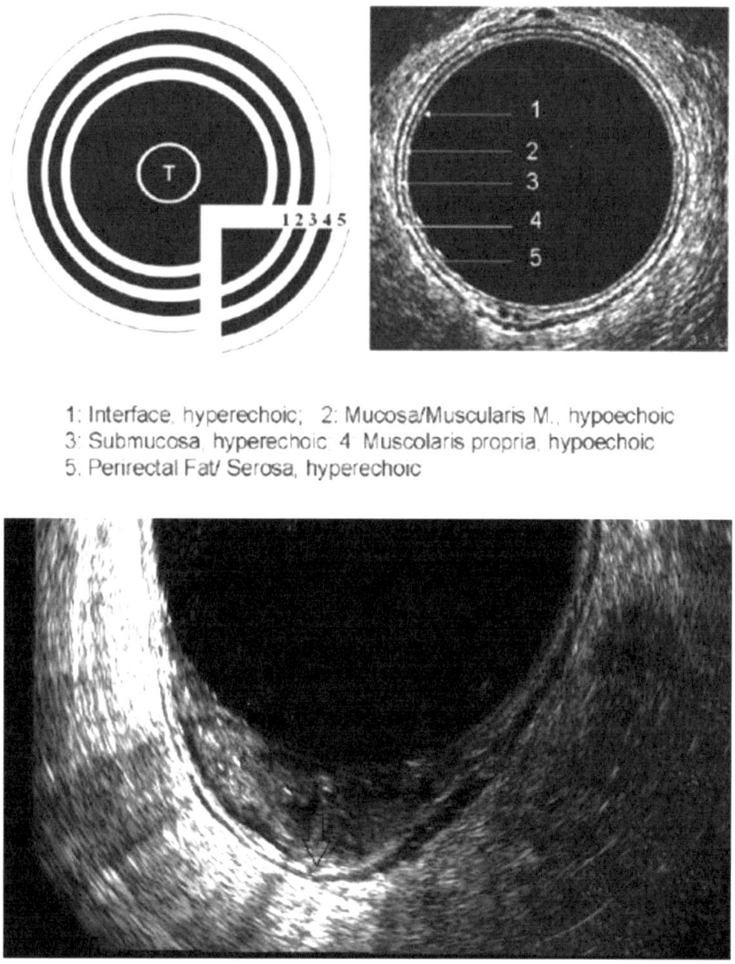

Figure 10. uT1 early polypoid tumor in lower rectum. Note the small breach in the submucosa (arrow) indicating tumor infiltration.

rectal walls must be fully distended to prevent wall folding and all captures must be done with a properly centralized probe in the perpendicular position, related to longitudinal rectal axis.

By using this technique, it is possible to address almost every rectal tumor at any height in a reliable and reproducible fashion (**Figures 12** and **13**).

However, it must be recognized that 3D EAUS has some limitations that may hinder adequate image capture or even prevent the exam completion.

First, when analyzing very small lesions one must be careful during rectal balloon distention. Whether excessive, such lesions could be compressed leading to tumor overstaging. Second, ulcerated lesions may create a gas-filled gap between lesion surface and the balloon, what is responsible for producing posterior acoustic shadows, impeding adequate perirectal fat evaluation or making the evaluation impossible in some situations. Third, stenosing tumors may prevent the exam simply by not allowing the probe to pass through the lesion up to proximal rectum [18].

Moreover, the examiner must be aware of two or more special situations that are worth mentioning: first, the inflammatory process shortly after the rectal cancer biopsy, could lead to T overstage and second, after neoadjuvant treatment, the inflammatory process caused by radiation only subsides in 55/60 days. An exam taken during this period is likely to be inaccurate in differentiating rectal layers and to overstage T or N status. In such cases, performing 3D EAUS at least 2 weeks after the endoscopic biopsy and roughly over 2 months after radio and chemotherapy completion is recommended [5].

Many studies have shown that 3D EAUS is comparable to MRI for T staging and in early rectal lesions, namely Tis-2 lesions; 3D EAUS is more accurate than MRI in identifying very small differences of compromised rectal walls layers. Albeit suboptimal, both methods are seemingly equivalent in accuracy regarding node status, although some authors have favored MRI [25–29].

When reporting pre-operative rectal cancer staging, the examiner must obligatorily fulfill some steps that encompass all information needed for proper stage lesions as well as for enabling comparison after neoadjuvant treatment [5, 26]. These steps are outlined below:

1. T staging
2. Percentage of rectal circumference involved by tumor
3. Axial, longitudinal measurements of the lesion
4. Mesorectal infiltrating extension
5. Distance from the most distal part of the lesion to the puborectal muscles
6. N stage (number and size)
7. Circumferential radial margin related to prostate or posterior vaginal wall
8. The prefix "u" must be added to the final report, ex.: final staging uT3 N0

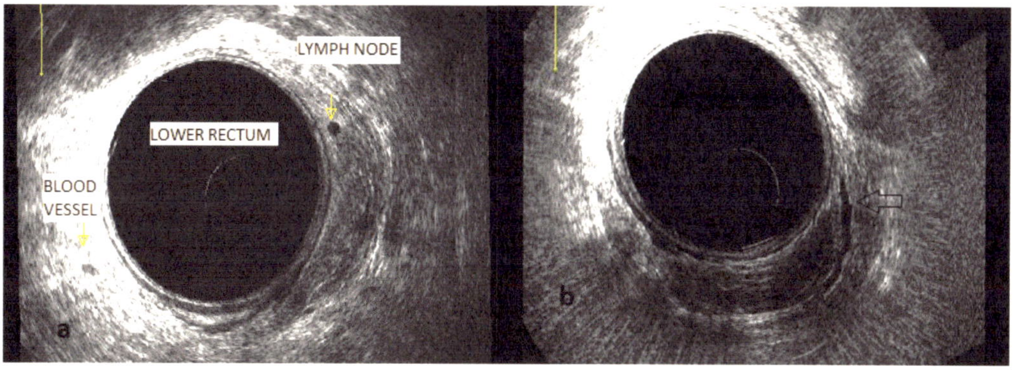

Figure 11. (a) Aspect of a lymph node in perirectal fat: hypoechoic, round-shape with regular borders (arrow). (b) In contrast, blood vessels appear as branch-like shape (arrows), in axial or sagittal views.

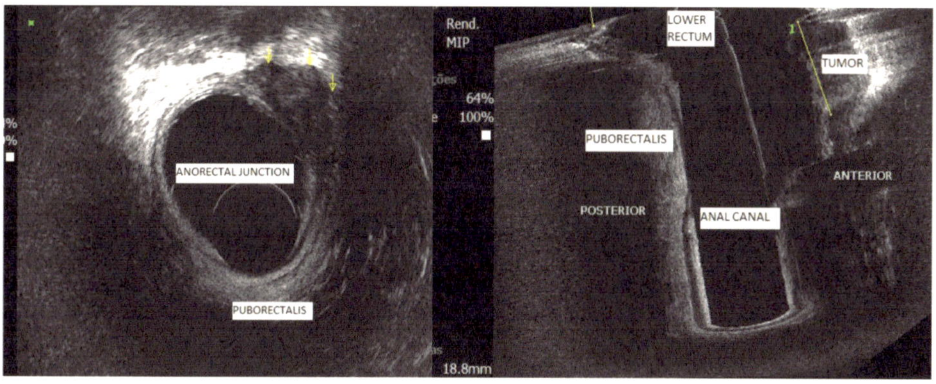

Figure 12. T3N0 tumor in lower rectum invading left puborectalis muscle. Axial view. Note the outer limits of the tumor infiltrating the perirectal fat (arrows). Sagittal/coronal view showing left anterolateral tumor locate at puborectalis level without invading intersphincteric plane.

3.2. Anal cancer

Anal cancers are rare lesions that correspond to less than 1% of all colorectal tumors. Anal canal tumors are more prevalent in women in their 5th–6th decades [30]. Despite radio/chemotherapy being the mainstay treatment of anal canal neoplasms, three-dimensional EAUS helps the surgeon in identifying sphincter or rectal involvement before treatment. Moreover, three-dimensional EAUS is capable of determining precise lesion measurement, identifying compromised perirectal or pelvic nodes or prostate/posterior vaginal wall invasion.

More importantly, three-dimensional EAUS is used to measure treatment response after radio/chemotherapy in order to discriminate cases for local excision, abdominoperineal resection or just follow-up with no organ resection instead. Furthermore, the presence of a well-delimited hypoechoic lesion identified 4–5 months after radio/chemo completion is very likely a tumor recurrence, needing excisional biopsy for confirmation [5, 31, 32].

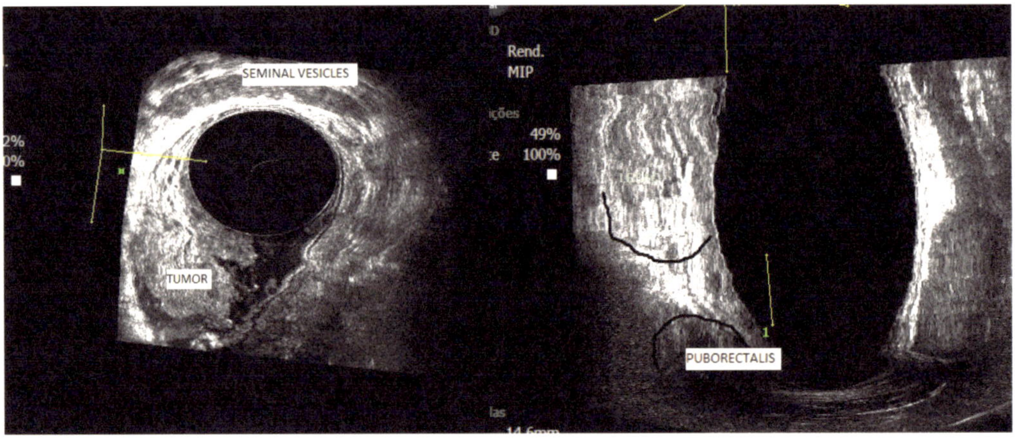

Figure 13. uT1N0 right lateral and posterior voluminous lateral spreading tumor (LST) in middle rectum. Left. Axial/coronal view: tumor spreads from seminal vesicles to the lower rectum. Right. Coronal view: lowest border located 1.5 cm proximal to the puborectalis muscle.

4. 3D EAUS dynamic scan ecodefecography

Constipation is a very common symptom with over 10% of patients reporting weekly episodes of difficult or obstructed evacuation in specialized centers. Despite considerable controversy on precise definition of constipation, recently published ROME IV criteria have separated constipation into two distinct types: inadequate defecatory propulsion and dyssynergic defecation [33]. Not rarely, some patients will present one or both types requiring more in-depth investigation.

Excluding extremely rare cases of colonic inertia, where a subtotal colectomy is required, surgical treatment of constipation will be reserved to patients with obstructed defecation which anatomical defects originate from dyssynergic pelvic floor symptomatic enough to justify surgical repair, mostly represented by anorectocele, internal intussusception or mucous and rectal prolapse or when associated with pelvic organ prolapse (POP).

Anorectal manometry, rectal balloon expulsion test, pudendal nerve latency test and defecography are complimentary techniques devised to assess the evacuation physiology and pathophysiology with arguable accuracy on reproducing such a dynamic and variable process [34].

Currently, 3D EAUS is a new adjunct technique that addresses dynamic pelvic floor motion during evacuation, in an ordered and reproductive fashion, comparable with defecography and better tolerated than MR defecography, without using radiation and taking no longer than 15 min [35, 36].

This novel modality known as echodefecography was devised by Murad-Regadas et al. in order to assess the middle/posterior pelvic compartment. It is capable of diagnosing occult sphincter defects, pelvic floor abnormal motion during straining, anismus, anorectocele, enterocele and anal/rectal prolapse. More recently, transvaginal scan was added to evaluate pubovisceral muscle injuries and urogenital hiatus measurement, as described below [37].

http://dx.doi.org/10.5772/intechopen.76620

The exam comprises four sequential scans:

Scan 1: Image acquisition is undertaken at rest to serve as reference for the normal position and measurement of pelvic muscles and organs.

Scan 2: The probe is inserted up to 6 cm. After 15 s at rest, the patient is asked to simulate an effort as during evacuation, sustained for 20 s.

Scan 3: The probe is inserted up to 7 cm until the anorectal junction is clearly viewed. After 15 s at rest, the patient is asked to simulate an effort as during evacuation, sustained for 20 s.

Scan 4: After rectal injection of 120 ml of US gel, image acquisition is set to the rectal scan mode. The probe is inserted up to 6 cm. After 15 s at rest the patient is asked to simulate an effort as during evacuation, sustained for 20 s [4].

In women with a history of vaginal delivery the measurement of the perineal body is routinely made in order to reveal occult sphincter injuries as well as guide surgeons in cases amenable to surgical repair of anterior/middle pelvic compartment prolapse. It is obtained by measuring the distance between the examiner's index finger held against posterior vaginal wall and the internal border of IAS in the middle anal canal (**Figure 14**).

4.1. Anismus

Anismus is diagnosed by gathering information from scans 1 and 3 as follows. At rest (scan 1) the angle formed between the line drawn parallel to the internal border of puborectalis muscle and the plane perpendicular to longitudinal axis of canal anal is measured.

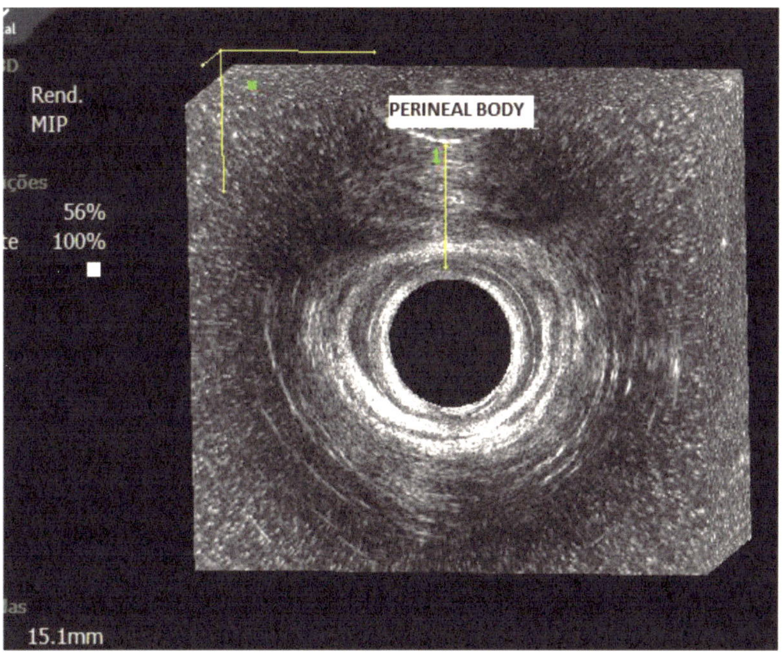

Figure 14. Normal perineal body thickness. Note the examiner index finger held against posterior vaginal all as reference. In women with no previous perineoplasty operation, measurement >10 mm is considered normal.

In scan 3, the angle is measured in the same way during straining. Normal puborectalis motion during straining occurs when the angle increases, suggesting that the muscle has moved away from the probe. In contrast, whether the angle narrows, indicating that the puborectalis muscle moves toward the probe, a diagnosis of animus can be made (**Figure 15**).

Albeit anismus is not amenable to surgical repair, we believe it should be addressed in symptomatic cases before surgical repair of initial pelvic organ prolapse or anorectocele; otherwise, surgical results can be compromised due to sustained strain during evacuation caused by a non-relaxing puborectalis muscle. Results of biofeedback training have shown improvement in over 60% of patients [38].

4.2. Anorectocele

The term anorectocele refers to the prolapse not from the rectal wall but rather from the anterior wall on the anorectal junction where the largest area of herniation lies. It can be identified and graded in scan 4 by measuring the distance between the posterior vaginal wall position at rest and the maximum distension observed during straining.

In normal conditions, the vaginal wall moves posteriorly compressing the anterior rectal wall and anal canal, during straining. When there is a defect in superior anal canal, the evacuation effort increases the rectal intra-luminal pressure forcing the vaginal wall forward, which creates herniation.

Likewise, the patient with the rectum filled with gel strains in order to expel the rectal content, simulating an evacuation effort. Whether an anterior defect in anorectal junction wall is present, one can easily identify the anorectocele herniation.

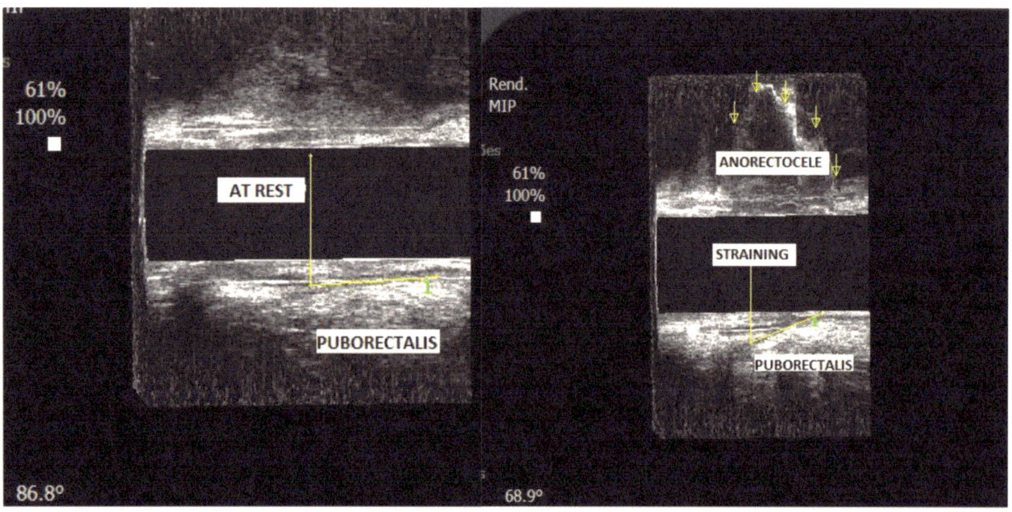

Figure 15. Left. Normal position of puborectalis muscle related to main anal canal axis, at rest. Right. Anismus and anorectocele. Decreased angle formed by the confluence of two lines drawn parallel to the internal border of puborectalis muscle and perpendicular to the anal canal axis, during straining. In anorectal junction (arrows), one can also note a grade III anorectocele.

Depending on the distance measured between the vaginal position at rest and the maximum herniation at straining, anorectocele can be graded as follows: grade I—up to 7 mm, grade II—7–13 mm and grade III—more than 13 mm or whether it exceeds the focal distance of the transducer. It is possible as well to visualize the herniation in axial planes (**Figure 16**).

Anorectocele could be present in 80% of adult population; most of them are asymptomatic, not requiring treatment. However, patients with external vaginal prolapse or with symptoms of rectal obstruction should be offered surgical repair, mostly cases with large anorectoceles (grades II and III). Recurrence, fecal urgency or incontinence and risk of dyspareunia must be thoroughly discussed with patients prior to surgery.

Colorectal surgeons usually prefer a transanal approach to treat anorectocele by using procedures such as stapled transanal rectal resection (STARR) specially devised to repair anorectocele plus internal rectal prolapse [39].

Even though STARR addresses these conditions simultaneously, anorectocele is frequently associated with other conditions as pelvic organ prolapse (POP), especially in older women; see Section 4.5. Peters et al. estimated that in women with rectal prolapse and obstructed defecation, over 60% had rectocele or occult rectal prolapse associated [40].

By using ecodefecography, we have observed that the majority of women with obstructed defecation have at least one anatomical pelvic floor abnormality. More importantly, occult rectal prolapse can mimic an anorectocele during a physical exam, therefore, misleading surgeons to unnecessary repair. 3D EAUS can easily depict anatomical and dynamic disturbances in posterior pelvic compartment, separating these two entities reliably. Besides, ecodefecography has very good correlation with defecography, is better tolerated by patients than MRI defecography and a total scan acquisition is no longer than 15 min, without using radiation (**Figure 17**).

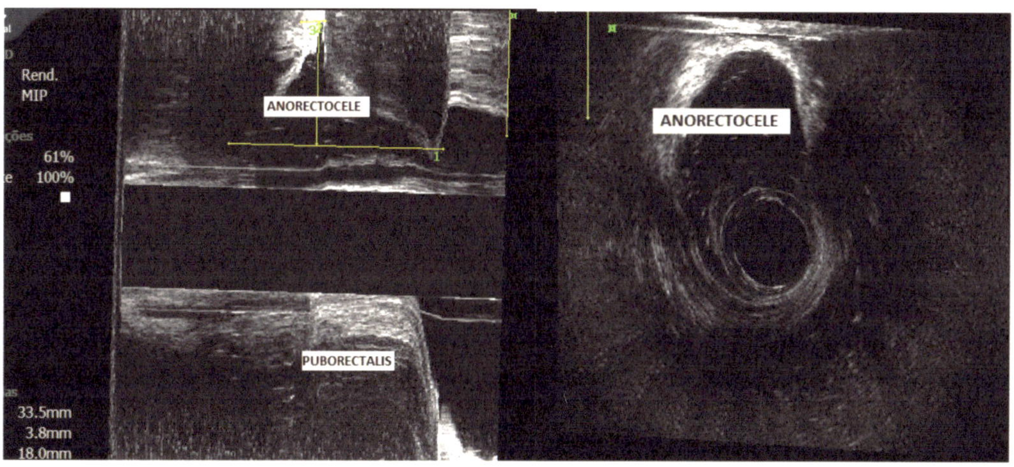

Figure 16. Patient with grade III (18.0 mm) anorectocele. Sagittal and axial views, image with gel.

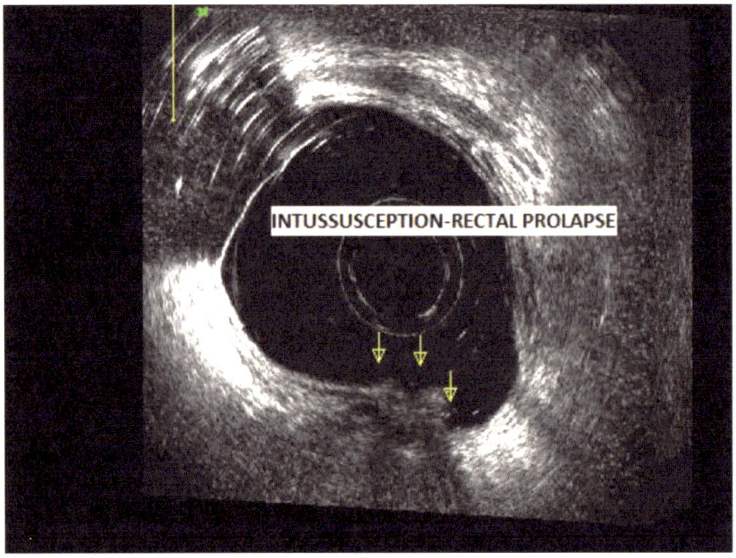

Figure 17. Posterior rectal prolapse. Rectal wall movement toward the lumen during straining (arrows).

4.3. Perineal descent

In all four scans previously described, probe position must follow the pelvic floor movement during straining, and the displacement of pelvic muscles is not taken into account. However, when measuring pelvic floor downward motion, we should add another scanning, this time keeping the probe static. By doing that, the probe will serve as a neutral reference allowing a reliable measurement of pelvic motion.

The transducer is introduced up to 5–6 cm until the puborectalis muscle is clearly visualized. Keeping the probe static, the capture is initiated and the patient is asked for continuously straining until the puborectalis muscle is visible again, when straining is stopped. Hence, this technique allows to quantify perineal descent movement by measuring the distance between the cranial border of puborectalis muscle at rest and at its final position, after completing an evacuation effort (**Figure 18**).

Perineal descent is not a surgically correctable disease. When associated with other correctable anatomical posterior compartment defects, we believe it must be treated prior to operation in order to not compromise surgical results, as in anismus [38].

4.4. Anal/rectal prolapse

Anal prolapse or mucous prolapse is diagnosed by measuring the thickness of the most internal layer that lies between the probe and IAS. Usually, a mucous prolapse can be diagnosed when the thickness measured is over 3 mm.

Rectal prolapse could be divided into overt rectal prolapse (rectal procidentia) and occult rectal prolapse (internal intussusception). Occult rectal prolapse is diagnosed in scan 3 and 4. During straining, one or multiple folds are observed toward rectal lumen. These images are better viewed in sagittal plane as double muscle layers, although it is not uncommon to identify internal intussusception in the axial plane as shown in **Figure 17**.

Internal intussusception can be diagnosed in asymptomatic patients. However, constipated patients with rectal prolapse, partial or circumferential, especially when associated with ano-rectocele, are good candidates to surgical repair, for example, by using a transanal approach to stapler rectopexy as described earlier [39].

Overt rectal prolapse is a self-evident condition, usually without needing any routine imaging exam. However, due to multi-compartment etiology of pelvic organ prolapse it is advisable to assess comprehensively the entire pelvic floor, especially in older women with symptoms of obstructed defecation or fecal incontinence, given in detail in the later section.

4.5. Pelvic organ prolapse

Patients with obstructed defecation, especially whether they have had childbirth trauma in the past, may evolve in the long term with anatomical anterior, middle or posterior compartment disorders on the pelvic floor muscle and endopelvic fascia, sometimes culminating in pelvic organ prolapse (POP) [41].

Frequently, dyssynergic pelvic floor or fecal incontinence is also present in this population so that colorectal surgeons pay close attention to that multi-compartment feature of the syndrome before surgical repair. Rather, the modern assessment of POP is now managed by a multidisciplinary team through female pelvic medicine reconstructive surgery (FPMRS) where the colorectal surgeon is a relevant part.

In some cases, history and physical examination are self-evident but routine a pelvic organ prolapse quantification (POP-Q) is used to measure and report prolapse (**Table 2**).

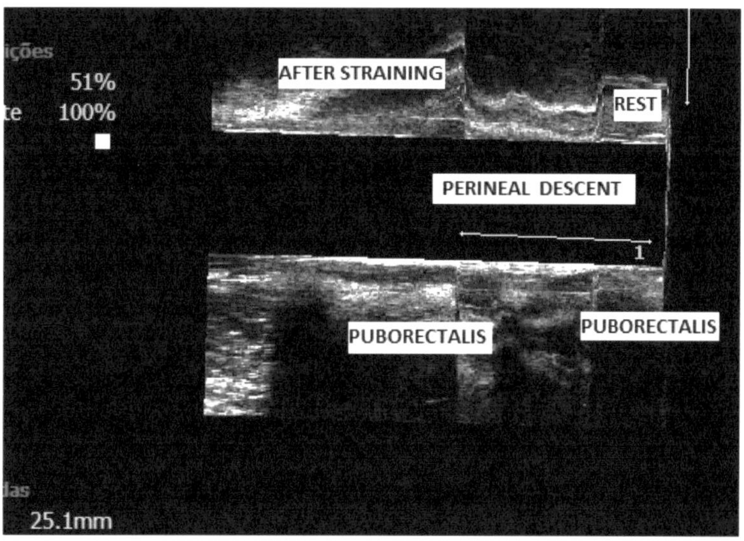

Figure 18. Patient with perineal descent. Puborectalis muscle displacement downward >2.5 cm after straining.

Stage 0	No prolapse; apex descends within 2 cm of the total vaginal length
Stage 1	Most distal portion of the prolapse descends to a point greater than 1 cm above the hymen
Stage 2	Most distal portion of the prolapse descends to a point within 1 cm above the hymen (above and below)
Stage 3	Prolapse extends more than 1 cm beyond the hymen but no more than within 2 cm of total vaginal length
Stage 4	Complete eversion; extension within 2 cm of the total vaginal length

Table 2. Pelvic organ prolapse stages.

Based on symptoms, the POP-Q stage and associated anatomical disorders, some cases may be candidates to surgical treatment [42]. Thus, due to the multi-compartmental nature of the disease, it is imperative before operation to obtain a comprehensive pelvic floor dynamic evaluation to define the best therapeutic planning.

Generally, patients without significant clinical response to conservative treatment and overt pelvic organ prolapse should be submitted to surgical repair. However, some cases are more defying and question the route to surgical approach, whether transvaginal or abdominal, need of colorectal resection or concomitant anti-incontinence procedure; they should all be considered with regard to the patient, in a pre-operative setting.

Pelvic ultrasonography has been used in order to evaluate POP, initially by transperineal bidimensional mode and recently, with modern software, 3D EAUS or even transperineal three-/four-dimensional reconstruction of pelvic images by tomography as pioneered by Dietz et al. [43] .

Recently, a transvaginal scanning has been added to the regular echodefecography exam, in order to address the pelvic floor muscle anatomy alongside the measurement of urogenital hiatus, mainly focusing on middle and posterior compartments [35–37].

The transvaginal scan is acquired in the rectal mode, using the same probe as in rectal capture, needing a rectal balloon attached to it. Usually, the transducer is introduced until the bladder

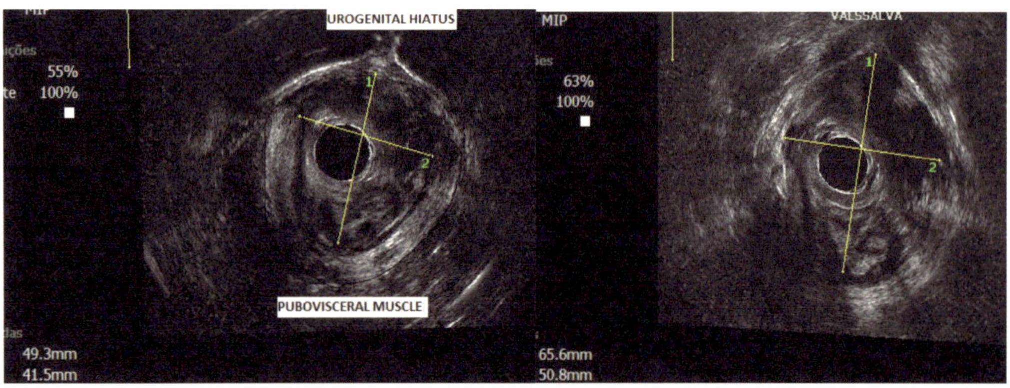

Figure 19. Left. Transvaginal scanning at rest, using the 3D endoanal probe. Detail of pubovisceral muscle. Right. Significant increase of urogenital hiatus during Valsalva maneuver indicating possible room for occult organ prolapse.

neck anteriorly is clearly visualized. A scan at rest and during Valsalva maneuver is sufficient to depict pelvic organs' position and integrity of the pubovisceral muscle bilaterally.

Bilateral pubovisceral muscle integrity is measured at rest paying special attention to its insertion on the pubic rami.

Biometric index of urogenital hiatus is obtained by measuring the anteroposterior diameter (distance between inferior margin of symphysis pubis and the inner margin of pubovisceral muscle) and laterolateral diameter (the distance between the inner margins of the lateral branches of the pubovisceral muscle at the level of their attachments to the pubic bone), at rest and after Valsalva maneuver (**Figure 19**).

Bladder neck position and anorectal junction position, related to the lower margin of symphysis pubis at rest and after Valsalva maneuver, are compared in order to measure pelvic organ motion [37].

Based on these findings, surgeons can define more accurately pelvic floor abnormalities in dubious cases, in those with unsatisfactory response to conservative therapy or after surgical repair of overt pelvic organ prolapse.

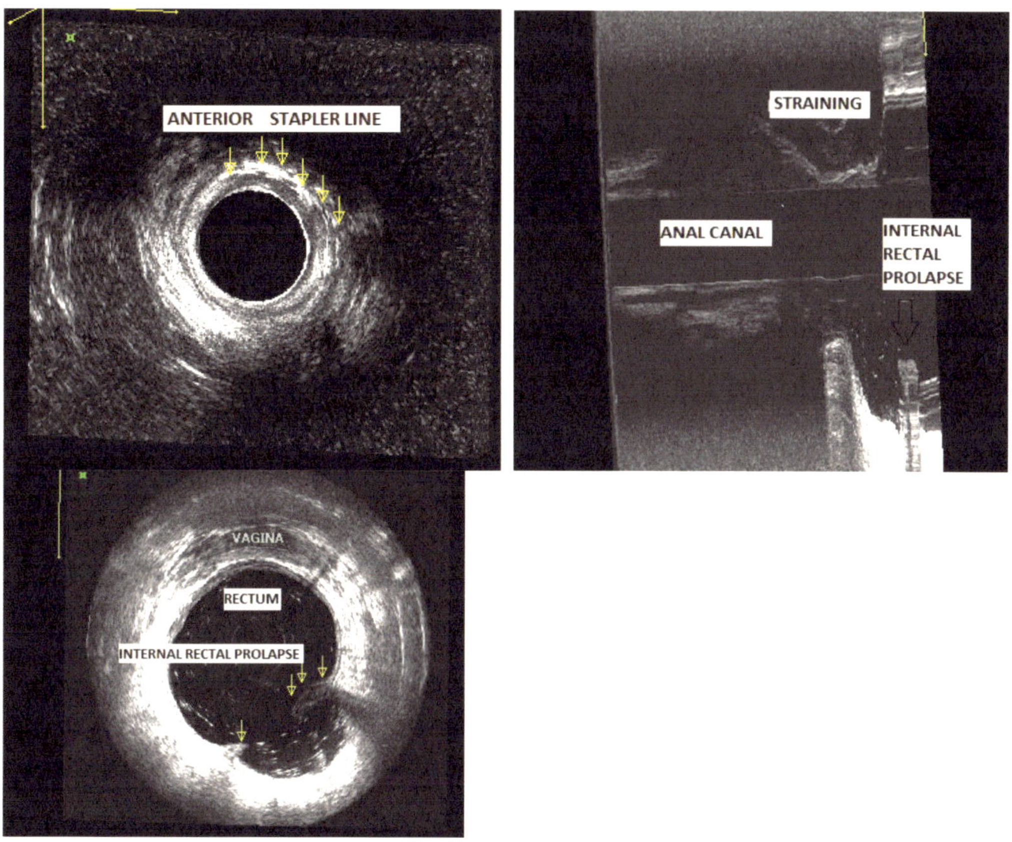

Figure 20. Upper left: axial plane. Anterior suture line after STARR for anorectocele repair. Upper right: Sagittal plane. Normal motion of the repaired posterior vaginal wall during straining. Down: Patient symptomatic for obstructed defecation after surgery due to an unsuspected occult rectal prolapsed not identified during physical examination.

Moreover, before surgical repair of anorectocele or occult rectal prolapse, for instance, echodefecography with transvaginal scanning is able to identify an unsuspected cystocele, an enterocele or sigmoidocele mimicking an anorectocele or even an abnormal anorectal junction motion during evacuation. This comprehensive assessment of the pelvic floor will certainly modify treatment planning.

On the other hand, in post-operative settings, ecodefecography is a suitable tool for evaluation in a reliable and reproducible way; successful surgical repair once is capable of measuring the improvement in pelvic floor abnormal motion, proper mesh position in case of POP surgery and finally the proper stapling line position after anorectocele repair (**Figure 20**).

5. Conclusion

In conclusion, 3D EAUS has now a well-established place in modern colorectal practice providing surgeons with valuable information in pre-operative and post-operative evaluation of patients with benign as well as malignant anorectal diseases and pelvic floor disorders. Conversely, 3D EAUS may benefit not only surgical but non-surgical cases as well, by adding relevant information unsuspected by clinical assessment alone.

We believe that 3D EAUS will keep on gaining ground in colorectal surgery, especially in benign anorectal diseases and pelvic floor evaluation. With the ongoing development of new software as modern transducers, we hope in the near future the exam could be more widespread in the colorectal community, overcoming its examiner-dependent limitation.

Acknowledgements

I would like to thank Dr. Stella Maria Murad-Regadas for the inspiring dedication to three-dimensional ultrasound and for all teaching after these long 10 years.

Conflict of interest

I declare no conflict of interest.

Author details

Marcelo de Melo Andrade Coura

Address all correspondence to: md.coura1@gmail.com

Colorectal Surgery Department, School of Medicine, Brasilia University Hospital, University of Brasilia, Brasilia, Brazil

References

[1] Law PJ, Bartram CI. Anal endosonography: Technique and normal anatomy. Gastrointestinal Radiology. 1989;**14**:349-353

[2] Abdool Z, Sultan AH, Thakar R. Ultrasound imaging of the anal sphincter complex: A review. The British Journal of Radiology. 2012;**85**(1015):865-875. DOI: 10.1259/bjr/27314678

[3] Regadas FSP, Murad-Regadas SM, Lima DMR, Silva FR, Barreto RGL, Souza MHLP, Regadas Filho FSP. Anal canal anatomy showed by three-dimensional anorectal ultrasonography. Surgical Endoscopy. 2007;**12**:2207-2211. DOI: 10.1007/s00464-007-9339-0

[4] Murad-Regadas SM, Regadas FSP, Rodrigues LV, Kenmoti VT, Fernandes GOS, Bunchen G, Regadas Filho FSP. Effect of vaginal delivery and ageing on the anatomy of the female anal canal assessed by three-dimensional anorectal ultrasound. Colorectal Disease. 2012;**14**(12):1521-1527. DOI: 10.1111/j.1463-1318.2012.03033.x

[5] Pescatori M, Regadas FSP, Murad Regadas SM, Zbar AP, editors. Imaging Atlas of the Pelvic Floor and Anorectal Diseases. 1st ed. Italy: Springer-Verlag; 2008. p 91. ISBN: 978-88-470-0808-3

[6] Steele SR, Kumar R, Feingold D, Rafferty JL, Buie WD. The standards practice task force, the American Society of Colon and Rectal Surgeons. Practice parameters for the treatment of perianal abscess and fistula-in-ano. Diseases of the Colon and Rectum. 2011;**54**:1465-1474. DOI: 10.1097/DCR.0b013e31823122b3

[7] Santoro GA, Fortling B. The advantages of volume rendering in three-dimensional endosonography of the anorectum. Diseases of the Colon and Rectum. 2007;**50**:359-368. DOI: 10.1007/s10350-006-0767-z

[8] Nagendranath C, Saravanan MN, Sridhar C, Varughese M. Peroxide-enhanced endoanal in preoperative assessment of complex fistula-in-ano. Techniques in Coloproctology. 2014;**18**(5):433-438. DOI: 10.1007/s10151-013-1067-y

[9] Toyonaga T, Tanaka Y, Song JF, et al. Comparison of accuracy of physical examination and endoanal ultrasonography for preoperative assessment in patients with acute and chronic anal fistula. Techniques in Coloproctology. 2008;**12**:217-223. DOI: 10.1007/s10151-008-0424-8

[10] Madbouly KM, El Shazly W, Abbas KS, Hussein AM. Ligation of intersphincteric fistula tract versus mucosal advancement flap in patients with high transsphincteric fistula-in-ano: A prospective randomized trial. Diseases of the Colon and Rectum. 2014;**57**:1202-1208. DOI: 10.1097/DCR.0000000000000194

[11] Siddiqui MR, Ashrafian H, Tozer P, Daulatzai N, Burling D, Hart A, et al. A diagnostic accuracy meta-analysis of endoanal ultrasound and MRI for perianal fistula assessment. Diseases of the Colon and Rectum. 2012;**5**:576-585. DOI: 10.1097/DCR.0b013e318249d26c

[12] Parks AG, Gordon PH, Hardcastle JD. A classification of fistula-in-ano. British Journal of Surgery. 1976;**63**(1):1-12

[13] Mellgren A. Fecal incontinence. Surgical Clinics of North America. 2010;**90**(1):185-194. DOI: 10.1016/j.suc.2009.10.006

[14] Markland AD, Goode PS, Burgio KL, et al. Incidence and risk factors for fecal incontinence in black and white older adults: A population-based study. Journal of the American Geriatrics Society. 2010;**58**(7):1341-1346. DOI: 10.1111/j.1532-5415.2010.02908.x

[15] Pescatori M, Favetta U, Dedola S, Orsini S. Transanal stapled excision of rectal mucosal prolapsed. Techniques in Coloproctology. 1997;**1**:96-98

[16] Sultan AH, Kamm MA, Hudson CN, Thomas JM, Bartram CI. Anal-sphincter disruption during vaginal delivery. New England Journal of Medicine. 1993;**329**:1905-1911

[17] Siegel R, Desantis C, Jemal A. Colorectal cancer statistics. CA: A Cancer Journal for Clinicians. 2014;**64**:104-117. DOI: 10.3322/caac.21220

[18] Marone P, Bellis M, D'Angelo V, et al. Role of endoscopic ultrasonography in the loco-regional staging of patients with rectal cancer. World Journal of Gastrointestinal Endoscopy. 2015;**7**:688-701. DOI: 10.4253/wjge.v7.i7.688

[19] Park J, Jang Y, Choi G, Park S, Kim H, Kang H, Cho S. Accuracy of preoperative MRI in predicting pathology stage in rectal cancers: Node-for-node matched histopathology validation of MRI features. Diseases of the Colon and Rectum. 2014;**57**:32-38. DOI: 10.1097/DCR.0000000000000004

[20] Beets-Tan RG, Lambregts DM, Maas M, Bipat S, Barbaro B, Caseiro-Alves F, et al. Magnetic resonance imaging for the clinical management of rectal cancer patients: Recommendations from the 2012 European Society of Gastrointestinal and Abdominal Radiology (ESGAR) consensus meeting. European Radiology. 2013;**23**:2522-2531. DOI: 10.1007/s00330-013-2864-4

[21] Monson JR, Weiser MR, Buie WD, Chang GJ, Rafferty JF, Buie WD, et al. Practice parameters for the management of rectal cancer (revised). Diseases of the Colon and Rectum. 2013;**5**:535-550. DOI: 10.1097/DCR.0b013e31828cb66c

[22] Habr-Gama A, Perez RO, Nadalin W, Sabbaga J, Ribeiro Jr U, Silva e Souza AHJ, et al. Operative versus nonoperative treatment for stage 0 distal rectal cancer following chemoradiation therapy: Long-term results. Annals of Surgery. 2004;**240**(4):711-717. DOI: 10.1097/01.sla.0000141194.27992.32

[23] Puli S, Bechtold M, Reddy J, Choudahary A, Antilles M, Brugge W. How good is endoscopic ultrasound in differentiating various T stages of rectal cancer? Meta-analysis and systematic review. Annals of Surgical Oncology. 2009;**16**:254-265. DOI: 10.1245/s10434-008-0231-5

[24] Hildebrandt U, Feifel G. Preoperative staging of rectal cancer by intrarectal ultrasound. Diseases of the Colon and Rectum. 1985;**28**:42-46. DOI: 10.1007/BF02553906

[25] Kim NK, Kim MJ, Yun SH, Sohn SK, Min J. Comparative study of transrectal ultrasonography, pelvic computerized tomography, and magnetic resonance imaging in

preoperative staging of rectal cancer. Diseases of the Colon and Rectum. 1999;**42**:770-775. DOI: 10.1007/BF02236933

[26] Garcia-Aguillar J, Pollack J, Lee SH, et al. Accuracy of endorectal ultrasonography in preoperative staging of rectal tumors. Diseases of the Colon and Rectum. 2002;**45**:10-15. DOI: 10.1007/s10350-004-6106-3

[27] Al-Sukhni E, Milot L, Fruitman M, Beyene J, Victor J, Schocker S, Brown G, McLeod R, Kennedy E. Diagnostic accuracy of MRI for assessment of T category, lymph node metastases, and circumferential resection margin involvement in patients with rectal cancer: A systematic review and meta-analysis. Annals of Surgical Oncology. 2012;**19**:2212-2223. DOI: 10.1245/s10434-011-2210-5

[28] Landman RG, Wong WD, Hoepfl J, Shia J, Guillem JG, Temple LK, Paty PB, Weiser M. Limitations of early rectal cancer nodal staging may explain failure after local excision. Diseases of the Colon and Rectum. 2007;**50**:1520-1525. DOI: 10.1007/s10350-007-9019-0

[29] Park J, Jang Y, Choi G, Park S, Kim H, Kang H, Cho S. Accuracy of preoperative MRI in predicting pathology stage in rectal cancer: Node-for-node matched histopathology validation of MRI features. Diseases of the Colon and Rectum. 2014;**57**:32-38. DOI: 10.1097/DCR.0000000000000004

[30] Simpson JAD, Scholefield JH. Diagnosis and management of anal intraepithelial neoplasia and anal cancer. BMJ. 2011;**343**:d6818. DOI: 10.1136/bmj.d6818

[31] Parikh J, Shaw A, grant LA, et al. Anal carcinomas: The role of endoanal ultrasound and magnetic resonance imaging in staging, response evaluation and follow-up. European Radiology. 2011;**21**:776-785. DOI: 10.1007/s00330-010-1980-7

[32] Otto SD, Lee L, Buhr HJ, et al. Staging anal cancer: Prospective comparison of transanal endoscopic ultrasound and magnetic resonance imaging. Journal of Gastrointestinal Surgery. 2009;**13**(7):1292-1298. DOI: 10.1007/s11605-009-0870-2

[33] Simren M, Palsson OS, Whitehead WE. Update on Rome IV criteria for colorectal disorders: Implications for clinical practice. Current Gastroenterology Reports. 2017;**19**:15-23. DOI: 10.1007/s11894-017-0554-0

[34] Azpiroz F, Enck P, Whitehead W. Anorectal functional testing: Review of collective experience. The American Journal of Gastroenterology. 2002;**97**:232-240

[35] Regadas FS, Haas EM, Abbas M, Jorge JM, Habr-Gama A, Sands D, Werner S, Melo-Amaral I, Sardinas C, Lima D, Sagae E, Murad-Regadas SM. Prospective multicenter trial comparing echodefecography with defecography in the assessment of anorectal dysfunction in patients with obstructed defecation. Diseases of the Colon and Rectum. 2011;**54**:686-692. DOI: 10.1007/DCR.0b013e3182113ac7

[36] Murad-Regadas SM, Regadas FS, Rodrigues LV, et al. A novel three-dimensional dynamic anorectal ultrasonography technique (echodefecography) to assess obstructed defecation, a comparison with defecography. Surgical Endoscopy. 2008;**22**:974-979. DOI: 10.1007/s00464-007-9532-1

[37] Murad-Regadas SM, Fernandes GOS, Regadas FSP, Rodrigues LV, et al. Assessment of pubovisceral muscle defects and levator hiatal dimensions in women with faecal incontinence after vaginal delivery: Is there a correlation with severity of symptoms? Colorectal Disease. 2014;**3**:1010-1018. DOI: 10.1111/codi.12740

[38] Patcharatrakul T, Gonlachanvit S. Outcome of biofeedback therapy in dyssynergic defection patients with and without irritable bowel syndrome. Journal of Clinical Gastroenterology. 2011;**45**:593-598. DOI: 10.1097/MCG.0b013e31820c6001

[39] Meurette G, Wong M, Frampas E, Regenet N, Lehur PA. Anatomical and functional results after stapled transanal rectal resection (STARR) for obstructed defecation. Colorectal Disease. 2011;**13**:e6-e11. DOI: 10.1111/j.1463-1318.2010.02415.x

[40] Peters WA, Smith MR, Drescher CW. Rectal prolapse in women with other defects of pelvic floor support. American Journal of Obstetrics and Gynecology. 2000;**184**:1488-1495. DOI: 10.1067/mob.2001.114853

[41] Varma M, Rafferty J, Buie WD. Standards practice task force of American Society of Colon and Rectum Surgeons. Practice parameters for the management of rectal prolapse. Diseases of the Colon and Rectum. 2011;**54**:1339-1346. DOI: 10.1097/DCR.0b013e3182310f75

[42] Lim M, Sagar PM, Gonsalves S, Thekkinkattil D, Landon C. Surgical management of pelvic organ prolapse in females: Functional outcome of mesh sacrocolpopexy and rectopexy as a combined procedure. Diseases of the Colon and Rectum. 2007;**50**:1412-1421. DOI: 10.1007/s10350-007-0255-0

[43] Dietz HP. Pelvic floor ultrasound: A review. Clinical Obstetrics and Gynecology. 2017;**60**(1):58-81. DOI: 10.1097/GRF.0000000000000264

Section 3

Rectal Prolapse

Chapter 4

Challenges in the Surgical Treatment of Rectal Prolapse

Renato Pietroletti

Additional information is available at the end of the chapter

http://dx.doi.org/10.5772/intechopen.78059

Abstract

The approach to a patient with overt rectal prolapse remains controversial since the choice of the most appropriate technical option may be a difficult task. The different approaches are based upon patients' age, comorbidities, sex, size of prolapse, associated incontinence, constipation, and urinary and genital disturbances. However, analysis of the literature failed to detect a significant evidence favoring one among the large number of those different surgical techniques proposed for the treatment of rectal prolapse. In fact, many randomized prospective controlled trials, comparing perineal and abdominal operations, rectopexy alone, resection alone and/or resection plus rectopexy could not find significant differences in terms of morbidity, mortality, improvement of incontinence or constipation, quality of life and recurrence. Therefore, without a clear-cut support by the literature, a pragmatic approach is necessary, applying common sense, experience and considering the availability of resources as well. Nevertheless, we may expect that definitive answers to many open questions about surgery of rectal prolapse may come from larger studies and longer follow-up.

Keywords: rectal prolapse, surgery, abdominal, perineal, procedure

1. Introduction

The complete prolapse of the rectum is a true intussusception of the viscus outside of the anus, through the sphincters. Aged multiparous women are mainly affected, even if earlier observations reported a significant incidence in nulliparous or psychiatric patients [1, 2]. In males, the rectal prolapse tends to appear in younger patients, but in any patient, a history of chronic constipation and excessive straining is reported. Some anatomical abnormalities represent predisposing factors of rectal prolapse and many other are a consequence of the prolapse itself [3]. Abnormally lax attachments of the rectum to the sacrum and to lateral pelvic walls, a deep

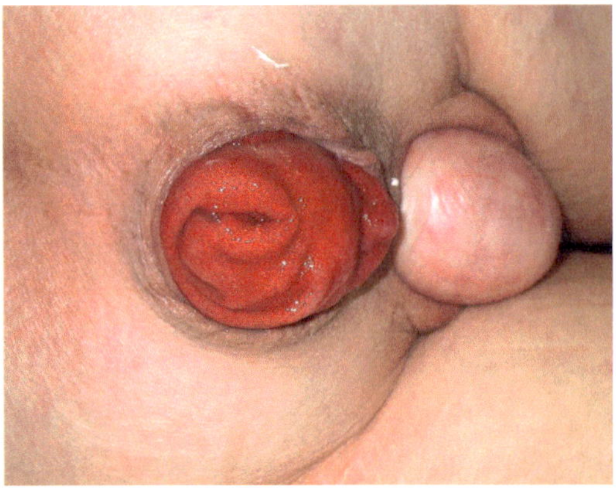

Figure 1. Complete prolapse of the rectum involving also mid-anterior compartments.

peritoneal pouch between rectum and vagina or bladder are invariably observed. Consequently, the long-standing stretching in pelvic structures will result in other associated abnormalities which affect also the anterior and middle compartments, depicting the so called "tetralogy of fall-out syndrome" (**Figure 1**). Genital prolapse, urinary incontinence, perineal descent, levator diastasis, patulous anus and finally pudendal nerve stretch with consequent neuropathy and anal sphincter weakness are frequently observed, either alone or in combination. The attempts to explain the etiology of rectal prolapse generated several different theories, all looking at one or more of the observed anatomical defects as the main abnormalities predisposing to rectal prolapse and thus proposing a specific surgical treatment. A typical example is represented by the theory of the sliding hernia by Moscowitz [4], who proposed the suturing of the deep pouch of Douglas as a targeted surgical therapy. Instead, the cineradiographic studies of Broden and Snelleman [5] identified the cause of rectal prolapse in a complete recto-rectal intussusception. In those patients complaining of chronic constipation (the vast majority), this symptom may be accompanied by impaired intestinal transit time, dolichocolon, redundant sigmoid colon or a true sigmoidocele. The latter one can be also the cause of a severe obstructed defecation. All these mentioned conditions may complicate and worsen the clinical picture of a complete rectal prolapse and must be taken into consideration, in planning surgical treatment.

Overt rectal prolapse is a disabling and embarrassing condition since the quality of life of the patient is marred by symptoms such as mucus discharge, true incontinence, bleeding, obstructed defecation and although rarely, pain. Not to mention the occurrence of complications such as massive bleeding, ischemia or incarcerated prolapse all requiring emergency abdominal surgery leading almost invariably to intestinal stoma.

2. Prolapse in children

Regardless of sex, rectal prolapse is reported rarely in children older than 3 years of age and is uncommon in western countries. The rectal prolapse in children is mostly due to either excessive straining at defecation or because of an acute respiratory disease [6] such as pertussis. Usually,

	Patients (no.)	Results (%)
Sclerosing injection	414	83–100
Anal encirclement	40	97–100
Presacral packing	100	100
Linear cauterization	73	97
Rectopexy	8	100

Table 1. Treatment results of rectal prolapse in children, data from the literature.

it is represented by a simple prolapse of rectal mucosa and conservative treatment has a great percentage of success, as soon as the children grow. In case of failure, different procedures could be indicated, the simplest one being represented by injection sclerotherapy. However, if surgical treatment is needed, we can rely upon a great number of different operations, similarly to an adult patient. **Table 1** summarizes different treatments and results in pediatric patients.

3. Complete rectal prolapse in adult

Kairaluoma [7] estimated the annual prevalence of rectal prolapse in the adult population in about 2.5/100.000 affecting more commonly women than men [8]. Childbirth, straining at stool, anatomical abnormalities and progressive laxity of rectal attachments, also related to menopausal, hormonal changes can represent etiologic factors and account for the increasing frequency of complete rectal prolapse observed with age progression in females. In males, on the contrary, the peak of incidence is around 30–40 years of age. As said earlier, following the cine-radiographic studies of Broden and Snelleman, the anatomical defect causing complete prolapse of the rectum is represented by a true recto-rectal intussusception. Among the other anatomical abnormalities, the observation of a deep peritoneal pouch, supporting early pathogenetic hypothesis of complete rectal prolapse being as a sliding hernia, is a complementary defect. Instead, this anatomical abnormality together with the pelvic floor deficiency, the genital descent and urinary disturbances, all represent a consequence of the continuous straining of the rectum. Therefore, apart from the occurrence of prolapse, not rarely the patient complains of many other symptoms of pelvic floor failure, the main one being fecal incontinence. Interestingly, continence improvement after surgical treatment of rectal prolapse is reported in up to 77% of the cases in the experience of various authors. [1–3, 8]

From the clinical point of view, the most common complaint is related to the presence of the prolapse itself, sometime reported as feeling of a balloon or a foreign body in the perineum. Tenesmus, mucous discharge, or true fecal incontinence, together with symptoms of obstructed defecation, almost invariably complete the clinical picture. If the prolapse is not appearing spontaneously, the patient must be asked to strain, either in the left lateral or in the squatting position. Alternatively, we could ask the patient to take a picture of the prolapse at its maximal descendent by himself using a smartphone. The author says that a lot of patients already found this method of reporting of such symptoms of friendly use (**Figure 2**).

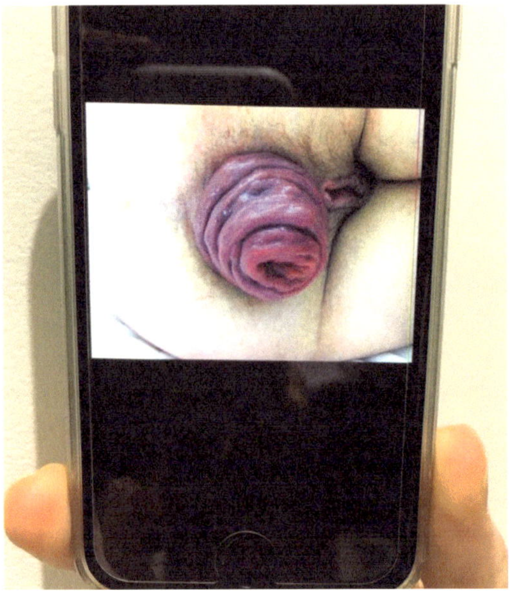

Figure 2. Self-reporting by a patient herself of rectal procidentia at maximum extent, with photograph.

As far as physical examination is concerned, a full thickness rectal prolapse will appear as a cylinder of bowel with its concentric, symmetric folds. Conversely, a simple mucosal prolapse appears with its irregular, mainly radiated mucosal folds. To confirm the diagnosis of full thickness rectal procidentia, it is mandatory to palpate accurately the prolapse; this is to be done with the thumb inserted in the lumen of the prolapsed bowel and the first and second fingers on the external aspect, firmly grasping the bowel wall. In this way, the double thickness of the prolapsing bowel is easily recognizable. At the same time, by means of gentle pressure, the rectum can be squeezed back and repositioned inside the pelvis.

Before surgical treatment is planned, a complete diagnostic screening is needed and should be addressed to investigate continence, colon and rectum imaging, associated organs prolapse. In patients with a reasonably long life expectancy, it is mandatory the control of any co-existing functional bowel disorder, since a complete anatomical cure of the prolapse is not to be counter-balanced by a poor quality of life, related to bad bowel function.

Colonoscopy is invariably needed to exclude other diseases also in view of patients' age. Anorectal manometry, although with its limitations, can be useful particularly when coupled with trans anal ultrasound, the latter aimed to detect sphincter lesions especially in a multiparous woman. In addition, one of the recently developed continence questionnaire with a scoring system can be of utmost importance for grading incontinence and for follow-up purposes [9, 10].

As for imaging studies, contrast enema may depict the redundant sigmoid colon and a multi-contrast proctography may detect the associated abnormalities of the pelvic floor. In this respect, pelvic MRI or MRI defecography [11] may replace, in expert hands, conventional radiographic studies, detecting at the same time the involvement of pelvic organs other than rectum [12] However, conventional multicontrast defecography appears superior in diagnosing rectocele or enterocele [13]. Radiographic transit time studies might be indicated in case of severe, longstanding constipation, in order to rule out delayed transit of the whole colon with consequent implications of surgical treatment.

The correlation between rectal prolapse and chronic psychiatric diseases has been often reported [1–3]. In recent years, such association became even more evident although ill-understood; autism [14] and other forms of behavioral abnormalities are often observed in rectal prolapse, contributing to poor outcome in case of surgical treatment [15, 16]. In addition, an emerging behavioral abnormality such as anorexia nervosa is found to be not rarely complicated by rectal prolapse [17]. All the spectrum of eating disorders, when coupled with laxative abuse, rectal purging, forced defecation and excessive straining may lead to overt rectal prolapse [18, 19]. Such aspects deserve a particular attention and they need to be fully evaluated before surgery is planned.

Finally, a few considerations are due to the complete prolapse of an ileal pouch. In the large experience of the Cleveland Clinic, pouch prolapse after ileo-anal procedure has been reported in 0.3% of the patients [20]. Since pouch surgery is becoming more and more popular, we might expect a rise in its incidence. **Figure 3** shows a complete prolapse of a pouch, in a patient after total proctocolectomy for complications of Hirschsprung disease. Treatment of this condition may be challenging and preferably conducted by means of abdominal, mesh pouch-pexy, however not rarely ending in pouch loss and permanent stoma [20, 21].

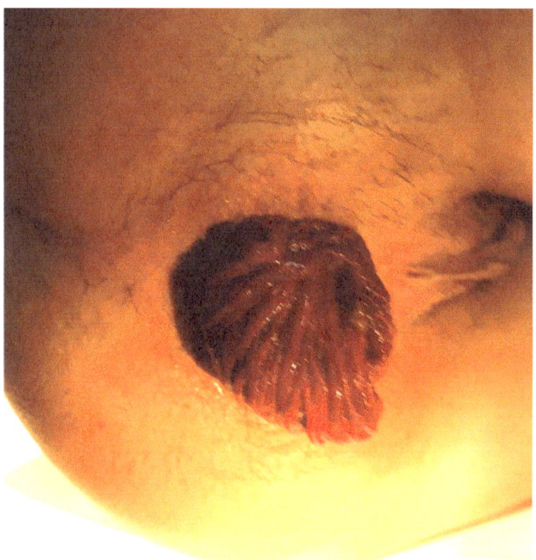

Figure 3. Complete prolapse of an ileal pouch.

4. Principles of surgical treatment

The history of the surgical treatment of rectal prolapse is rich of several, different surgical techniques, all proposed with the aim of eliminating the anatomical defect which was believed to be the main responsible for the prolapse. According to Kuijpers [22], the literature reports a list of authors who proposed to treat the prolapse by means of different techniques; encircling the anus, or plicate or resect the prolapse, or to suspend and/or fix it or to wrap with foreign material.

Such wide variability of surgical approach may be related to the leading theory born in the mind of the surgeon about the pathogenesis of the prolapse; the strong believe in a specific anatomical defect of pelvic floor as the main responsible of the rectal prolapse, represented the milestone suggesting the development of targeted operations, each focused on that anatomical abnormality. In addition, different categories of patients were encountered in clinical practice as far as age, sex, associated illnesses is concerned. They need a personalized treatment, especially in terms of low morbidity/mortality and less invasive procedures for an aged and risky patient. In recent times however, the full understanding of rectal prolapse pathophysiology has eliminated the debate around several, obsolete surgical procedures, practically abandoned. Nonetheless, still some controversial issues exist on a handful of operations commonly performed, referring in particular to the choice of abdominal versus perineal approach. In the vast majority of cases, we are approaching complete rectal prolapse in a geriatric patient with associated illnesses, not rarely in the ASA status III or IV; only a small amount of individuals is represented by a young patient, in good physical conditions. In addition, we should take into account that the various anatomical defects accompanying (not causing!) rectal prolapse need to be treated anyway, possibly at the same time; last but not least, we must pay attention to all the associated symptoms (fecal incontinence, constipation, urinary incontinence, sexual disturbances), planning treatment and adequate follow-up in an "holistic" approach.

We may conclude that the ideal surgical treatment for correction of the rectal prolapse should be mini-invasive, with low morbidity, almost nihil mortality and a reasonable percentage of recurrence.

Due to the clinical characteristics of majority of the patients, as mentioned earlier, it is not surprising that perineal procedures have been developed and became quite popular with respect to more invasive abdominal operations. Therefore, the choice is debated between abdominal approach and perineal procedure taking into consideration factors other than age and performance status of the patient.

5. Perineal operations

The simplest contenitive treatment of the rectal prolapse was represented by a suture encircling the anus. The original procedure was that one proposed by Tiersch (**Figure 4**), encircling the anus with a wire. Other modifications of the original technique involved the use of different material such as silicone, mesh, silastic rings or Angelchik prosthesis. Results are poor

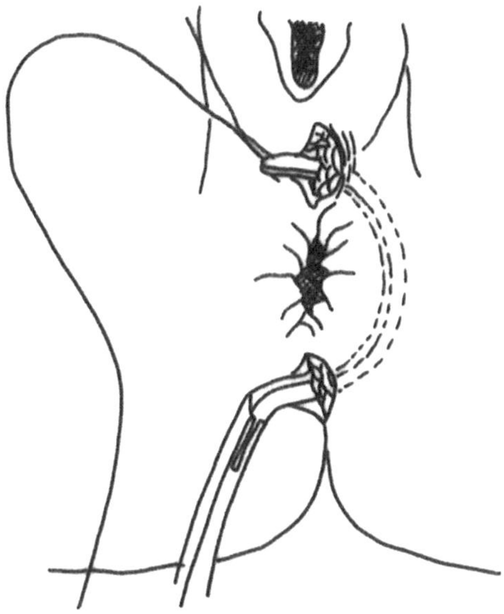

Figure 4. The anal encirclement procedure according to Tiersch.

and complications are frequent therefore these methods have been abandoned and herein are reported for completeness.

Edmonde Delorme, a French military surgeon, described the procedure of prolapse mucosectomy and plication of rectal wall [23]. The procedure is not invasive and becomes quite popular especially in Europe with good result in terms of morbidity, mortality and recurrence (**Table 2**).

Deaths are rarely reported, postoperative morbidity is represented mainly by bleeding, anal stricture may be observed as late sequelae. Recurrence varies between 5 and 26% with a mean value of 12–15%. Interestingly, adding a pelvic floor repair to Delorme's operation improves results in terms of continence and recurrence [24]. Our policy is to perform posterior levatorplasty routinely after a Delorme's procedure [25] with the aim of restoring a correct anorectal angle [26], increasing the height of the anal canal. This sort of anatomical restoration contributes to improve continence and reduces recurrence in our experience. In a recent study by Youssef [27], patients with rectal prolapse were randomly assigned to Delorme's operation or Delorme plus levatorplasty. The author reported improved continence and less recurrence in the group treated with levatorplasty respect to Delorme alone, thus confirming the rationale of levatorplasty as a fundamental tool in improving clinical results of Delorme's. This is confirmed in a retrospective, long-term follow-up study showing 9.9% actuarial incidence

No. of pts.	Mortality (%)	Recurrence (%)
414	0–1.2	5–26

Table 2. Results of Delorme's operation: cumulative data from the literature.

of prolapse recurrence. The absence of levatorplasty and the presence of constipation represented the risk factors [28].

The operation is carried out in lithotomy position, either in spinal or even local anesthesia. After infiltration of prolapsed rectum submucosa with diluted adrenaline (1:250,000 w/v) or epinephrine, the mucosa is stripped off starting 1 cm away from the dentate line, to the apex of the prolapse. Accurate hemostasis of rectal wall is achieved by diathermy. Following this, the rectal wall is plicated similarly to a concertina, by means of six to eight (The author prefers eight) longitudinal sutures taking four to five bites of rectal wall and then tied. The plicated prolapse is repositioned and the operation is terminated by suturing proximal rectal mucosa to the dentate line. As stated earlier, the posterior levatorplasty completes the procedure. The procedure is outlined in **Figures 5–10**.

This operation represents the ideal surgical treatment for those patients unfit for other more invasive procedures. Even if recurrence rate is not negligible, the operation is repeatable with a high chance of success [29] (**Table 3**).

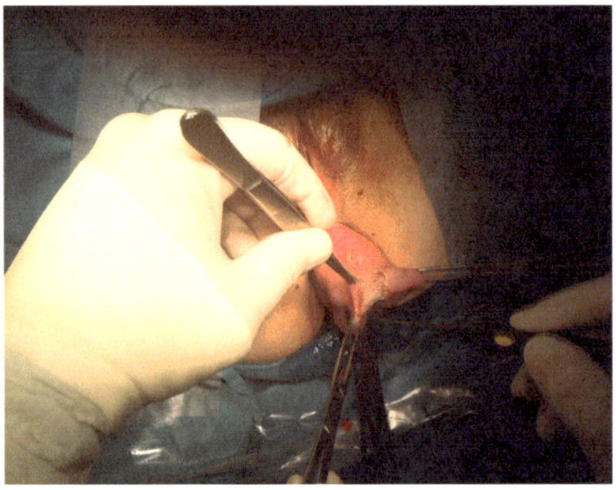

Figure 5. Mucosectomy of the rectal prolapse.

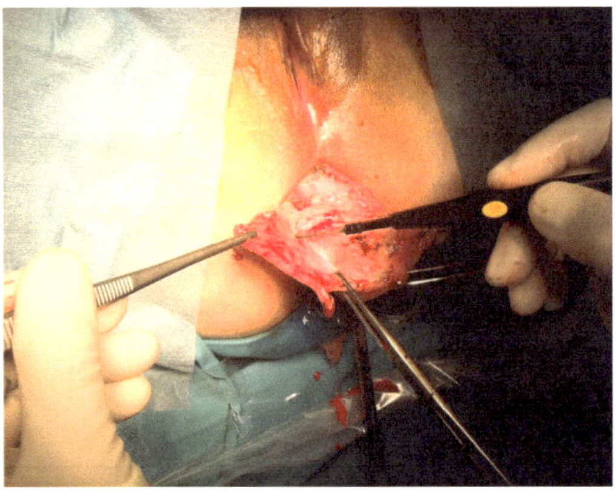

Figure 6. Mucosectomy is carried out by diathermy with careful hemostasis.

http://dx.doi.org/10.5772/intechopen.78059

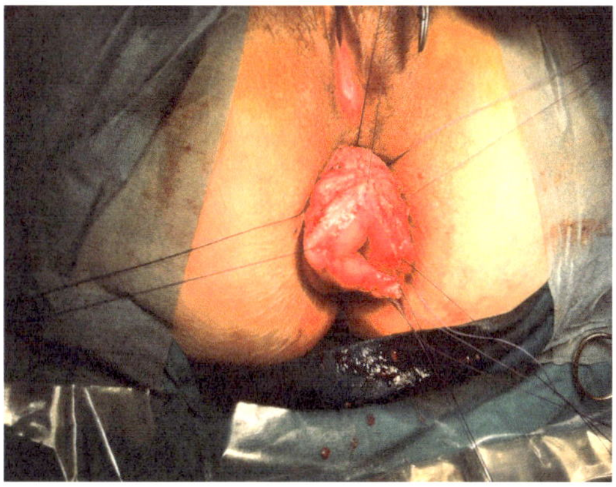

Figure 7. Plication of the prolapse with longitudinal sutures.

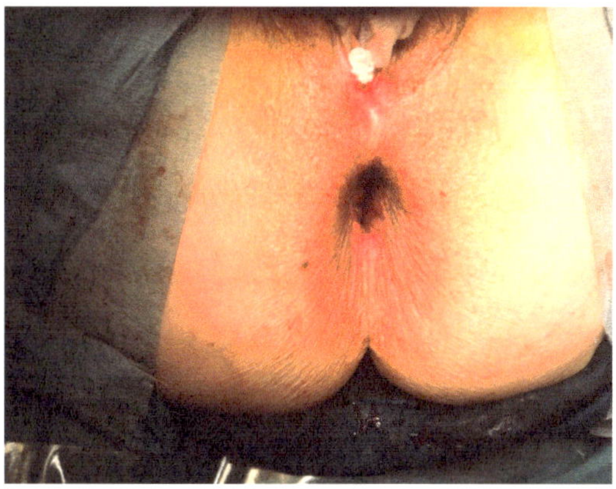

Figure 8. Patulous anus at the end of the procedure.

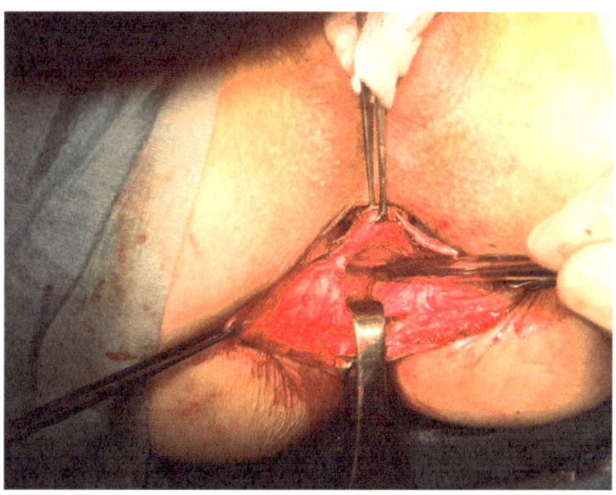

Figure 9. The two branches of levator muscles are identified for levatorplasty.

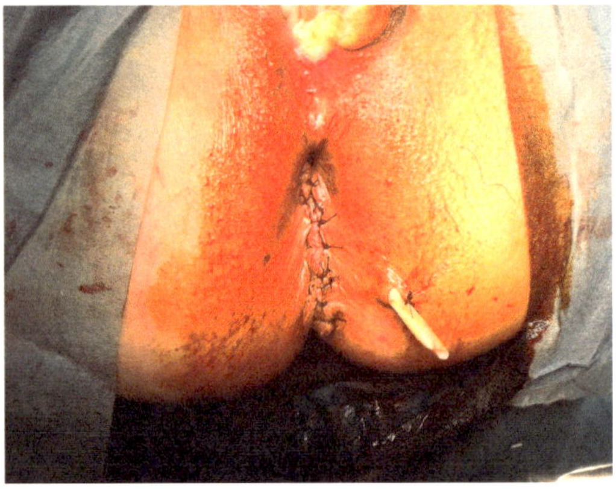

Figure 10. Posterior levatorplasty restores correct ano-rectal angle.

		Mortality	Morbidity	Recurrence	Improved continence	Comments
No. of pts	▪ 62					3 males
Median age	78 years (27–92)					1 pouch prolapse
Delorme	▪ 46	0	1*	3	28**	* Minor bleeding
	▪Associated levatorplasty in 26					** 26 delorme + levatorplasty
Resection rectopexy	12	0	2 ^	0	12	^ Sub-occlusion
Rectopexy	1	0	0	1	0	
Total	59 operated pts.°	0	3	4	40	° 2 pts. and 1 pouch prolapse operated elsewhere

Table 3. Surgery of complete rectal prolapse—author's personal experience.

Perineal rectosigmoidectomy was firstly described by Altemeier [2]. The procedure combines different advantages but also shows some weak points. In first place, the prolapsed rectum is excised, the deep peritoneal pouch is shortened and closed and finally, pelvic floor muscles can be repaired. It is therefore attractive to achieve such an extensive anatomical correction by means of a perineal operation, in a patient considered unfit for major abdominal surgery. Coming to the weak points however, recurrence is still a problem with its incidence varying from 3–43% [3, 8]. Moreover, incontinence may persist due to the loss of reservoir function following rectal resection. The operation can be performed in lithotomy or jack-knife positions, in spinal or preferably under general anesthesia with complete muscle relaxation. The rectal prolapse is attracted outside of the anus and a full thickness cut is made transversely at the level of the dentate line. The sigmoid colon is delivered through the incised peritoneum of the deep pouch of Douglas, the sigmoid vessels in the mesentery ligated and divided and then the proximal section of the prolapse is accomplished. At this time, the muscle fibers of the levator ani become evident anteriorly and may be plicated. Subsequently, the posterior aspect of the prolapse is approached and having divided the rectal wall, the mesorectum and puborectal sling become apparent. At this stage, plication of the puborectal muscle can be easily performed and after ligation of mesorectal vessels the prolapsed rectum with distal sigmoid colon is removed. The anastomosis between the resected proximal sigmoid and the dentate line is performed with interrupted sutures. Technical principles are depicted in **Figure 11**.

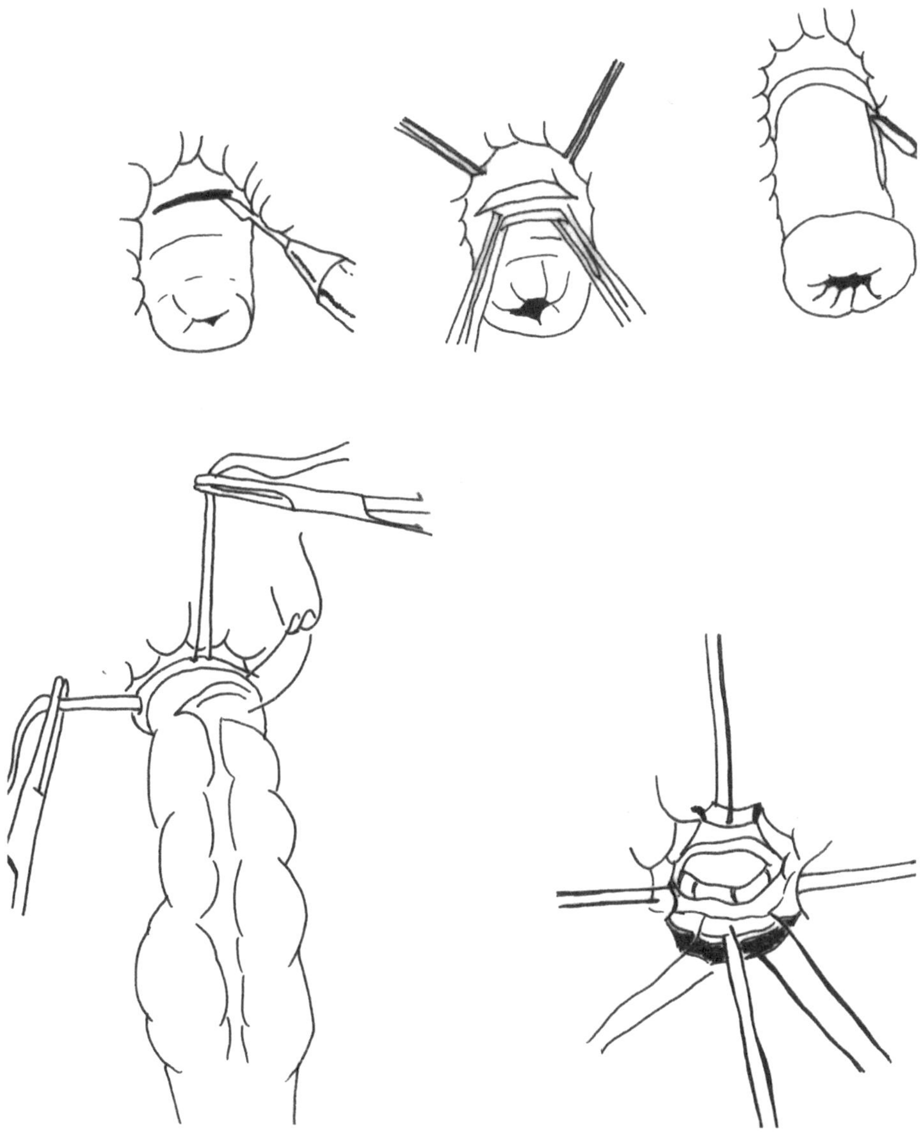

Figure 11. The Altemeier procedure depicted through the main stages.

No. of pts.	Mortality (%)	Recurrence (%)
738	0–6	0–50

Table 4. Results of Altemeier operation: cumulative data from literature.

In the case of Altemeier procedure too, in the experience of various authors, the pelvic floor repair improves the results of the operation either in terms of continence and recurrence rate [30, 31]. Modifications of the original technique include the use of mechanical circular stapler for the coloanal anastomosis, and the fashioning of a colonic pouch [8, 32]. In addition, pouch proctosigmoidectomy too showed to be superior to conventional Altemeier operation in terms of functional results (**Table 4**).

Pelvic floor repair alone and perineal rectopexy have to be mentioned among the perineal procedures employed for the treatment of rectal prolapse. However, they have been completely abandoned since their results showed to be very disappointing [8].

6. Abdominal procedures

Whenever possible (i.e. young, fit patients) an abdominal procedure should be preferred for treating rectal prolapse, in view of overall better results. The abdominal approach allows to treat the main defect simultaneously with other anatomical abnormalities. In fact, full mobilization of the rectum and fixation to the sacrum leaving lateral ligaments, thus preserving rectal innervation, guarantees from further intussusception. In addition, a deep peritoneal pouch can be repaired together with levator diastasis and should colonic resection be indicated, it may be easily accomplished via a laparotomic/laparoscopic approach. Not to mention the possibility of treating uterine or vaginal prolapse, bladder descent or anomalies of urethrovesical angle. Finally, the abdominal approach does not preclude the possibility of combining a perineal operation when needed; for instance, in presence of a large rectocele or vaginal prolapse a colpoperineorraphy or rectocele repair are easily approached from below.

All the abdominal procedures carry a slightly higher morbidity and mortality with respect to perineal operations, thus selection criteria are of utmost importance, considering the benign nature of the disease. In a propensity matched cohort of patients with comparable surgical risk status, no differences were found in terms of morbidity and mortality between perineal and abdominal operations [33], thus the progresses in anesthesiology, surgical techniques and technology and postoperative care make abdominal approach rather safe even in risky patients [34, 35].

6.1. Abdominal rectopexy

To date, little doubt exists in considering abdominal rectopexy as the gold standard in treating rectal prolapse in view of the very low (less than 2%) recurrence rate. The debate is rather moved on to the method of fixation (absorbable/non-absorbable suture, mesh of foreign material), the position of the mesh on the rectum (anterior, posterior), the fixation of the mesh (posterior or lateral) and finally whether or not a colonic resection should be performed.

http://dx.doi.org/10.5772/intechopen.78059

The earlier method of anterior rectopexy was that one developed by Ripstein [36] who attached the rectum after full mobilization, to the promontory of the sacrum by means of a sling of foreign material passing anteriorly (**Figure 12**), with the aim of fixing the rectum by a dense fibrous reaction. Not surprisingly the consequent scar tissue encircling the rectum was responsible for the development of stricture and obstructive complications (7–17%) and/or intractable constipation in up to 43% of the cases [3, 8]. Interestingly, Scaglia [37] reported a far low incidence of postoperative constipation when preserving lateral ligaments during rectal mobilization. As said earlier, leaving the rectal innervation untouched, by means of careful preservation of lateral attachments, guarantees a normal rectal sensation and therefore risks of postoperative constipation can be minimized.

Recently D'hoore [38] developed a new method of anterior rectopexy which seems to obviate the troubles of the Ripstein rectopexy. The rectum is mobilized and the dissection is deepened anteriorly. A mesh is then sutured to the anterior rectal wall and tractioned up in order to be fixed to the promontorium of the sacrum. Closure of the peritoneum completes the procedure (**Figure 13**). Results of this interesting type of anterior rectopexy, performed laparoscopically in the vast majority of the cases, or even with the help of robotic surgery are reported in **Table 5** and are quite encouraging [39, 40].

However also in this case, similarly to other comparative studies, results from a randomized protocol comparing laparoscopic, ventral mesh recto-pexy and Delorme's operation, failed to obtain significantly better results of one procedure over the other [41].

Some technical aspects are emerging from the literature and deserve consideration; in a female patient, the deep anterior dissection of the rectum from the vagina does not carry particular risks.

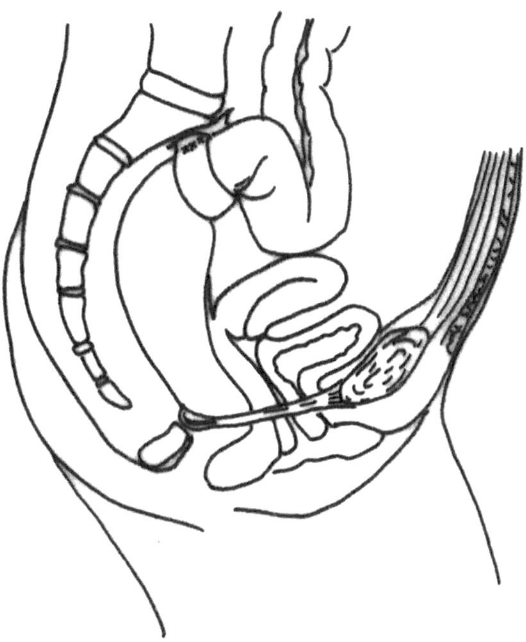

Figure 12. The Ripstein procedure, with the prosthesis anchoring the rectum anteriorly.

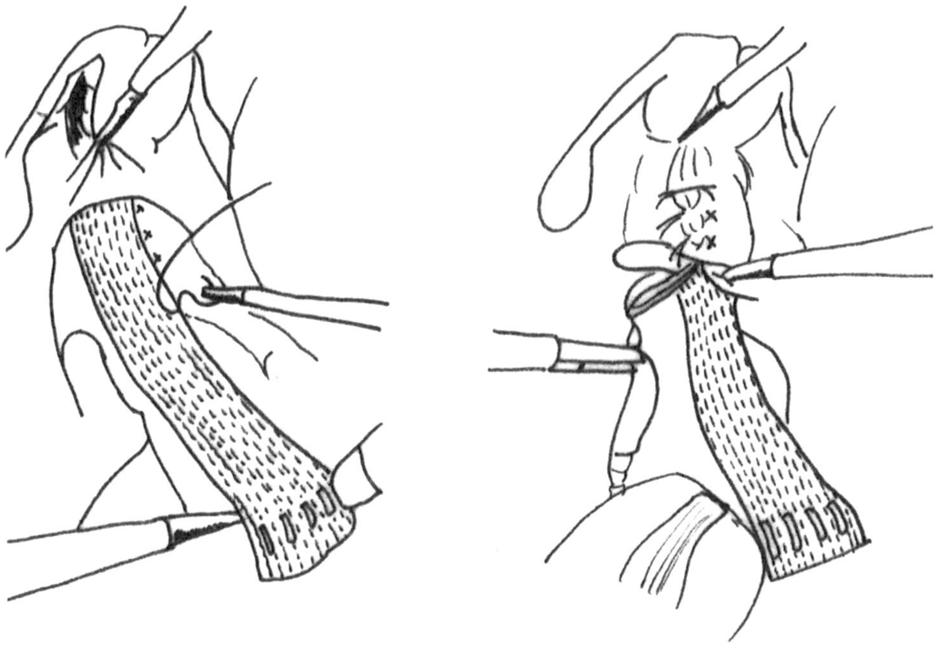

Figure 13. Laparoscopical suturing of the mesh on the anterior face of the rectum; peritoneization concludes the procedure.

n. of patients	251
Mean age	68 years
Follow-up	19–42 months
Mortality	0%
Morbidity	0–23.5%
Recurrence	2–5.8%
Improvement of incontinence	>80%
Improvement of constipation	>80%

Table 5. Cumulative data from literature of results in laparoscopic ventral mesh rectopexy (LVR).

In a male however, the deep anterior dissection of the rectum from seminal vesicles and prostate may be more challenging and even if it seems to be safe in terms of incidence of postoperative complications such as sexual disturbances (impotence, retrograde ejaculation) [42], unwilling problems in a young patient, reoperation rate has been reported to be not negligible [43], with 33% further surgery either due to persistent or recurrent prolapse. Other concerns may arise as far as mesh use in rectal surgery and in fact a new type of postoperative morbidity has been observed in case of ventral mesh rectopexy, that is mesh erosion. Evans reported 2% mesh erosion treated by mesh removal [44]. Borie also treated by means of mesh removal, the 7 patients complaining of mesh erosion out of 149 treated with laparoscopic ventral mesh rectopexy [45]. He found no worsening of functional symptoms. In conclusion, although of limited incidence and good prognosis, mesh erosion is a problem to be dealt with in case of laparoscopic ventral mesh rectopexy.

6.2. Resection and rectopexy

Resection alone gained a certain popularity, especially in the USA [46, 47] but the debate must be addressed to two main aspects, strictly correlated: in first place, it seems that in order to obtain adequate cure and low recurrence rate, the colon resection has to be wide, such as true anterior resection of the rectum with all the well-known technical difficulties not rarely encountered in such a demolitive operation (blood supply after ligation of inferior mesenteric artery, full mobilization of splenic flexure). This originates consequently, serious concerns about morbidity and mortality due to anastomotic and general complications; 3.5% mortality and 50% rate of septic complications are thrilling enough to move the majority of surgeons to a safer operation other than anterior resection, when a resective procedure is indicated.

Resection-rectopexy is also known as the Frykman-Goldberg [48] operation and is a sigmoid resection with sutured rectopexy to the sacrum (**Figure 14**).

There are strong evidences that this operation may be a very good choice for a young, fit patient [49]. In fact, it cures the prolapse with a very low recurrence, does not worsen incontinence, improves constipation, and allows the correction of other pelvic floor anomalies at the same time (**Table 6**).

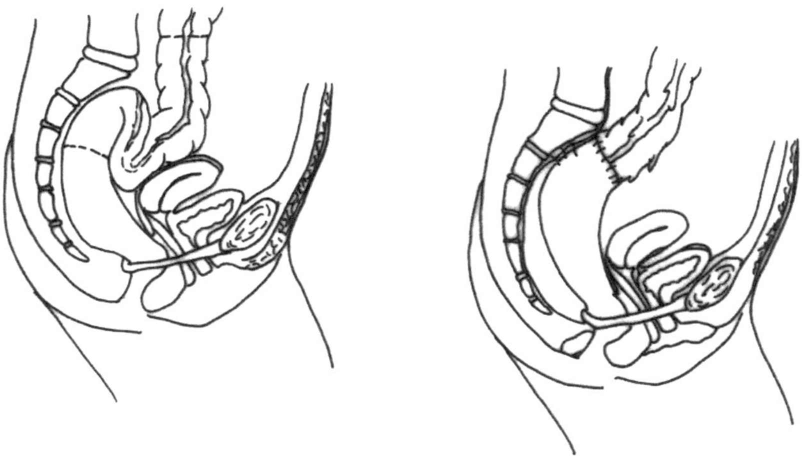

Figure 14. Sigmoid resection and sutured rectopexy according to the standard technique.

n. of patients	360
Mortality	0.8–2%
Morbidity	0–23%
Recurrence	0–9%
Improvement of incontinence	>85%
Improvement of constipation	>90%

Table 6. Cumulative data from literature of results in resection-rectopexy.

Since constipation, either in term of its persistency or "de novo" occurrence represents a major concern, leading to bad quality of life and probably being responsible for recurrence of prolapse, it is obviously attractive the idea of eliminating such problem with a safe resection such as a sigmoidectomy combined with rectopexy. A large amount of data from literature are now supporting the evidence that rectopexy alone might be responsible for severe post-operative constipation.

7. Choice of the best surgical option

Given so many variables in patient's selection, the best surgical option is still a case by case choice, highly dependent on surgeon's discretion and experience. In general, if the prolapse is short, not more than 4–5 cm up to 6–7 cm, the choice of a perineal operation is reasonable. Whereas in case of large prolapse measuring 10–15 cm it seems advisable an abdominal approach, preferably resection rectopexy. Unfortunately, if we search in the literature for supporting evidence, we cannot obtain conclusive data. In fact, in the last 20 years, two Cochrane systematic reviews were unable to draw any significant conclusion comparing different surgical techniques for the treatment of complete rectal prolapse [50, 51]. The final comment of the authors was that quality of papers was low, number of patients was inadequate and several methodologic bias were present. In a well-designed multicenter trial, the PROSPER trial, Senapati [52] tried to give answers to many open questions of surgical treatment of complete rectal prolapse. 340 patients were randomized to abdominal or perineal operation and subsequently each group further randomized to rectopexy alone or resection-rectopexy and Delorme's or Altemeier procedures. Quite surprisingly, no differences were found among all the compared operations; incidence of recurrence was similar between abdominal and perineal operations and even between Delorme and Altemeier and rectopexy versus resection/rectopexy. Also in all the other parameters investigated (morbidity, mortality, incontinence, constipation, quality of life), no operation showed to be superior to the others.

Another interesting contribution, come from an international survey by Formjine and Wexner [53]; surgeons from Europe and the USA were asked, by means of a detailed questionnaire, to indicate the preferred choice for rectal prolapse treatment. 391 surgeons from 50 different countries answered and results showed a sort of geographic dichotomy. In case of a high-risk patient the preferred approach was perineal for the majority of surgeons with a little prevalence of Delorme's operation in Europe with respect to the USA where Altemeier operation is more popular. As far as young patients are concerned, the different approach resulted quite sharp, with the USA more favorable for resection rectopexy and Europeans devoted to the newly developed ventral mesh rectopexy. This difference may be explained with the recent limitations of FDA for the use of prosthetic material in pelvic surgery, particularly in urogynecologic use. Quite interestingly a similar duality is observed also for internal rectal prolapse causing obstructed defecation. When operation is indicated, resection rectopexy is the choice of American surgeons, whereas in Europe the stapled transanal rectal resection (S.T.A.R.R. and Tran-S.T.A.R.R.) is favored. Also in this case, the recommendation concerning the risk of potentially severe complications of the two mentioned procedures, particularly in nonspecialist settings, prompted a prudent approach among American surgeons [54, 55].

8. Recurrent prolapse

The same principles applied for the treatment of complete rectal prolapse, can be employed for successful treatment of recurrences. Dedicated surgeons have to be familial with the approach to recurrent rectal prolapse since its incidence is not negligible, especially when a perineal operation is performed. Unfortunately, data from the literature do not give substantial support to the surgeon [56]. However, recent studies seem to indicate that resection rectopexy results in less than 10% recurrence rate [57], the progress in intra and postoperative care make resection rectopexy safe even in high-risk patients and we must consider that the literature reports a nearly 100% success for the treatment of recurrent prolapse [58]. But then, how can we select the right operation in case of recurrent rectal prolapse? The high chances of success of surgical treatment for recurrent rectal prolapse make us hypothesize that changing of surgical strategy, could address more properly to the right operation, perhaps that one probably indicated at the beginning. However, in case of recurrence, the adoption of the same operation previously performed is not to be disregarded. At the start, an intelligent question to ask to ourselves is related to the blood supply of the remaining bowel. In fact, all those patients who have undergone resection anastomosis may develop ischemia in case of a secondary resection. A good option in case of re-do operation for recurrent prolapse, especially if the length of the prolapsed bowel is no more than 4–5 cm and in presence of a risky patient can be the Delorme's plication. This operation in fact leaves untouched the main arterial flow to the rectum. However, if a suture rectopexy was the former choice, this can be repeated and better accompanied by a sigmoid resection. Steele [59] found in a very large study, that abdominal operations are associated with the lowest incidence of re-recurrence, when treating recurrent rectal prolapse and therefore this should be a preferred choice whenever possible. As a matter of fact, considering the benign nature of the disease, re-do abdominal surgery might be demanding both for the surgeon and the patient. Thus, we may conclude that an abdominal operation has to be considered in case of recurrence if previous operation was fixation rectopexy; if this is the case resection rectopexy is advisable. The same approach is to be considered if recurrent prolapse is more than 5–7 cm and the previous operation was a Delorme. On the contrary, if a repeated Delorme is not successful a third plication procedure can be safely repeated and probably, at this stage, the rectum is shortened enough to be suspended by its vascular pedicle. Obviously, in case of a repeated Delorme operation, it seems wise to add posterior levatorplasty.

9. Conclusions

Treatment of complete rectal prolapse remains a surgical dilemma. The complex picture of a full-thickness rectal prolapse needs to be approached in specialized centers, with the adequate case-load of patients. This means that surgical experience and a good amount of common sense are mandatory in order to plan a tailored surgical strategy. The right choice of the most appropriate operation must take into account all the associated anatomical modifications of pelvic floor. Chronic straining at defecation and/or constipation are invariably present in patients with rectal prolapse and thus every effort is to be addressed in investigating such symptoms and treat them. That's why preoperative investigations must be performed with the aim of detecting delayed intestinal transit, voiding disturbances, sexual troubles, mid compartment anomalies, fecal incontinence, nonrelaxing puborectal muscle. We must take into account that the persistence of a malfunctioning of the bowel will lead to failure of prolapse surgery and poor quality of life. On the other hand, once rectal prolapse is corrected, undertreatment of urogenital anomalies will lead to worsening of their symptoms. For old, risky patients, Delorme operation seems a straightforward approach coupled with posterior levatorplasty with the aim of reducing recurrence and improving continence. Recently, Cavazzoni [60], in a very preliminary study, proposed the implant of Gatekeeper prosthesis after Delorme operation with the aim of improving continence. Those patients with better physical performance are managed preferably by means of an abdominal operation also performed laparoscopically. Many surgeons are adopting laparoscopic, anterior mesh rectopexy, especially in Europe, whereas resection rectopexy remains popular in the USA. The first procedure faces the criticism of mesh erosion and high reoperation rate, especially in male patients, whereas the latter represents a gold standard in terms of low incidence of recurrence and good functional results. In addition, we should consider that due to the improvement of anesthesiology and patient's postoperative care, the standard sigmoid resection with sutured rectopexy can be proposed reasonably also in the older patient. In future, the wider diffusion of robotic surgery [61] may lead to the increasing use of such mini-invasive surgical technique also in abdominal surgery for complete rectal prolapse, with the aim of improving further the results.

Author details

Renato Pietroletti[1,2]*

*Address all correspondence to: renato.pietroletti@cc.univaq.it

1 Department of Clinical and Biotechnological Sciences, University of L'Aquila, AQ, Italy

2 Unit of Surgical Coloproctology, Hospital Val Vibrata, Sant'Omero, TE, Italy

References

[1] Goligher JC. Surgery of the Anus, Rectum and Colon. 5th ed. London: Bailliere-Tindall; 1984

[2] Altemeier WA, Cuthberson WR, Schowengerdt C, Hunt J. Nineteen years experience with the one stage perineal repair of rectal prolapse. Annals of Surgery. 1971;**173**:993-1006

[3] Keighley MRB, Williams NS. Rectal Prolapse in Surgery of the Anus, Rectum and Colon. 2nd ed. London: WB Saunders; 2007. pp. 794-842

[4] Moscowitz AV. The pathogenesis, anatomy and cure of prolapse of the rectum. Surgery, Gynecology & Obstetrics. 1912;**15**:7-21

[5] Broden B, Snelleman B. Procidentia of the rectum studied with cineradiography: A contribution to the discussion of causative mechanism. Diseases of the Colon and Rectum. 1968;**11**:330-347

[6] Greenberg DP, Von Konig CH, Heininger U. Health burden of pertussis in infant and children. Pediatric Infectious Disease Journal. 2005;**24**(suppl 5):S49-S43

[7] Kairaluoma MV, Kellokumpu IH. Epidemiologic aspects of complete rectal prolapse. Scandinavian Journal of Surgery. 2005;**94**(3):207-210

[8] Mills S. Rectal prolapse. In: Beck DE, Roberts PL, Saclarides TJ, Senagore AJ, Stamos MJ, Wexner SD, editors. The ASCRS Textbook of Colon and Rectal Surgery. 2nd ed. New York: Springer; 2011. pp. 549-563

[9] Jorge JM, Wexner SD. Etiology and management of fecal incontinence. Diseases of the Colon and Rectum. 1993;**36**:77-97

[10] Rockwood TH, Church JM, Fleshman JW, Kane RL, Mavrantonis C, Thorson AG, Wexner SD, Bliss D, Lowry AC. Fecal incontinence quality of life scale: Quality of life instrument for patients with fecal incontinence. Diseases of the Colon and Rectum. 2000;**43**(1):9-16

[11] Piloni V, Tosi P, Vernelli M. MR-defecography in obstructed defecation syndrome (ODS): Technique diagnostic criteria and grading. Techniques in Coloproctology. 2013 Oct;**17**(5):501-510. DOI: 10.1007/s10151-013-0993-z Epub 2013 Apr 5

[12] Lalwani N, Moshiri M, Lee JH, Bhargava P, Dighe MK. Magnetic resonance imaging of pelvic floor dysfunction. Radiologic Clinics of North America. 2013;**51**:1127-1139

[13] van Iersel JJ, Formijne Jonkers HA, Verheijen PM, Broeders IA, Heggelman BG, Sreetharan V, Fütterer JJ, Somers I, van der Leest M, Consten EC. Comparison of dynamic magnetic resonance defaecography with rectal contrast and conventional defaecography for posterior pelvic floor compartment prolapse. Colorectal Disease. 2017 Jan;**19**(1):O46-O53. DOI: 10.1111/codi.13563

[14] Van Heest R, Jones S, Giacomantonio M. Rectal prolapse in autistic children. Journal of Pediatric Surgery. 2004 Apr;**39**(4):643-644

[15] Hill SR, Ehrlich PF, Felt B, Dore-Stites D, Erickson K, Teitelbaum DH. Rectal prolapse in older children associated with behavioral and psychiatric disorders. Pediatric Surgery International. 2015;**31**(8):719-724. DOI: 10.1007/s00383-015-3733-9

[16] Marceau C, Parc Y, Debroux E, Tiret E, Parc R. Complete rectal prolapse in young patients: Psychiatric disease a risk factor of poor outcome. Colorectal Disease 2005 Jul;**7**(4):360-365

[17] Dreznik Z, Vishne TH, Kristt D, Alper D, Ramadan E. Rectal prolapse: A possibly underrecognized complication of anorexia nervosa amenable to surgical correction. International Journal of Psychiatry in Medicine. 2001;**31**(3):347-352

[18] Guerdjikova AI, O'Melia A, Riffe K, Palumbo T, McElroy SL. Bulimia nervosa presenting as rectal purging and rectal prolapse: Case report and literature review. The International Journal of Eating Disorders. 2012 Apr;**45**(3):456-459. DOI: 10.1002/eat.20959. Epub 2011 Aug 31. Review

[19] Mitchell N, Norris ML. Rectal prolapse associated with anorexia nervosa: a case report and review of the literature. Journal of Eating Disorders. 2013 Oct 10;**1**:39. DOI: 10.1186/2050-2974-1-39. eCollection 2013

[20] Joyce MR, Fazio VW, Hull TT, Church J, Kiran RP, Mor I, Lian L, Shen B, Remzi FH. Ileal pouch prolapse: Prevalence, management, and outcomes. Journal of Gastrointestinal Surgery. 2010 Jun;**14**(6):993-997. DOI: 10.1007/s11605-010-1194-y

[21] Changchien EM, Griffin JA, Murday ME, Bossart PW. Mesh pouch pexy in the management of J-pouch prolapse. Diseases of the Colon and Rectum. 2015 Apr;**58**(4):e46-e48. DOI: 10.1097/DCR.0000000000000337

[22] Kuijpers JHC. Treatment of complete rectal prolapse: To narrow, to wrap, to suspend, to fix, to encircle, to plicate or to resect? World Journal of Surgery. 1992 Sep-Oct;**16**(5):826-830

[23] Delorme E. Sur le traitement des prolapses du rectum totaux par l'escission de la muqueuse rectale ou rectocolique. Bulletin et Mémoires de la Société des Chirurgiens de Paris. 1900;**26**:499-518

[24] Lechaux JP, Lechaux D, Perez M. Results of Delorme's procedure for rectal prolapse: Advantages of a modified technique. Diseases of the Colon and Rectum. 1995;**38**:301-307

[25] Pietroletti R, Cianca G, Maggi G, Leardi S, Simi M. Trattamento chirurgico del prolasso del retto: interventi per via perineale. In: Proceedings of the 98° Congress of Societa' Italiana di Chirurgia; 13-18 October 1996; Rome Pozzi. pp. 397-411

[26] Kujipers JHC, de Morree H. Towards a selection of the most appropriate procedure in the treatment of complete rectal prolapse. Diseases of the Colon and Rectum. 1988;**31**:355-357

[27] Youssef M, Thabet W, El Nakeeb A, Magdy A, Alla EA, El Nabeey MA, Fouda El Y, Omar W, Farid M. Comparative study between Delorme operation with or without post-anal repair and levatorplasty in treatment of complete rectal prolapse. International Journal of Surgery. 2013;**11**(1):52-58. DOI: 10.1016/j.ijsu.2012.11.011

[28] Placer C, Enriquez-Navascués JM, Timoteo A, Elorza G, Borda N, Gallego L, Saralegui Y. Delorme's procedure for complete rectal prolapse: A study of recurrence patterns in the long term. Surgery Research and Practice. 2015;**2015**:920154. DOI: 10.1155/2015/920154

[29] Tobin SA, Scott IHK. Delorme operation for rectal prolapse. The British Journal of Surgery. 1994;**81**:1681-1684

[30] Friedmann R, Mugga-Sullam M, Freund HR. Experience with the one stage perieneal repair of rectal prolapse. Diseases of the Colon and Rectum. 1983;**26**:789-791

[31] Ramanujam PS, Venkatesh KS, Fiets MJ. Perineal excision of rectal procidentia in elderly, high-risk patients. Diseases of the Colon and Rectum. 1994;**37**:1027-1039

[32] Yoshioka K, Ogunbiyi OA, Keighley MRB. Pouch perineal recto-sigmodectomy gives better functional results than conventional recto-sigmoidectomy in elderly patients with rectal prolapse. The British Journal of Surgery. 1998;**85**:1525-1526

[33] Mustain WC, Davenport DL, Parcells JP, Vargas HD, Hourigan JS. Abdominal versus perineal approach for treatment of rectal prolapse: comparable safety in a propensity-matched cohort. The American Surgeon. 2013;**79**(7):686-692

[34] Laubert T, Bader FG, Kleemann M, Esnaashari H, Bouchard R, Hildebrand P, Schlöricke E, Bruch HP, Roblick UJ. Outcome analysis of elderly patients undergoing laparoscopic resection rectopexy for rectal prolapse. International Journal of Colorectal Disease. 2012 Jun;**27**(6):789-795. DOI: 10.1007/s00384-011-1395-1

[35] Clark CE 3rd, Jupiter DC, Thomas JS, Papaconstantinou HT. Rectal prolapse in the elderly: trends in surgical management and outcomes from the American College of Surgeons National Surgical Quality Improvement Program database. Journal of the American College of Surgeons. 2012;**215**(5):709-714. DOI: 10.1016/j.jamcollsurg.2012.07.004

[36] Ripstein CB. Procidentia: Definitive corrective surgery. Diseases of the Colon and Rectum. 1972;**15**:334-336

[37] Scaglia M, Fasth S, Hallgren T, Nordgren S, Oresland T, Hultén L. Abdominal rectopexy for rectal prolapse. Influence of surgical technique on functional outcome. Diseases of the Colon & Rectum. 1994 Aug;**37**(8):805-813

[38] D'Hoore A, Penninckx F. Laparoscopic ventral recto (colpo) pexy for rectal prolapse: Surgical technique and outcome for 109 patients. Surgical Endoscopy. 2006 Dec;**20**(12):1919-1923

[39] Faucheron JL, Trilling B, Girard E, Sage PY, Barbois S, Reche F. Anterior rectopexy for full-thickness rectal prolapse: Technical and functional results. World Journal of Gastroenterology. 2015 Apr 28;**21**(16):5049-5055. DOI: 10.3748/wjg.v21.i16.5049

[40] Faucheron JL, Trilling B, Barbois S, Sage PY, Waroquet PA, Reche F. Day case robotic ventral rectopexy compared with day case laparoscopic ventral rectopexy: A prospective study. Techniques in Coloproctology. 2016 Oct;**20**(10):695-700. DOI: 10.1007/s10151-016-1518-3. Epub 2016 Aug 17

[41] Emile SH, Elfeki HA, Youssef M, Farid M, Wexner SD. Abdominal rectopexy for the treatment of internal rectal prolapse: A systematic review and meta-analysis. Colorectal Disease. 2017 Jan;**19**(1):O13-O24. DOI: 10.1111/codi.13574

[42] Owais AE, Sumrien H, Mabey K, McCarthy K, Greenslade GL, Dixon AR. Laparoscopic ventral mesh rectopexy in male patients with internal or external rectal prolapse. Colorectal Disease. 2014 Dec;**16**(12):995-1000. DOI: 10.1111/codi.12763

[43] Rautio T, Mäkelä-Kaikkonen J, Vaarala M, Kairaluoma M, Kössi J, Carpelan-Holmström M, Salmenkylä S, Ohtonen P, Mäkelä J. Laparoscopic ventral rectopexy in male patients with external rectal prolapse is associated with a high reoperation rate. Techniques in Coloproctology. 2016 Oct;**20**(10):715-720. DOI: 10.1007/s10151-016-1528-1 Epub 2016 Sep 19

[44] Evans C, Stevenson AR, Sileri P, Mercer-Jones MA, Dixon AR, Cunningham C, Jones OM, Lindsey I. A multicenter collaboration to assess the safety of laparoscopic ventral Rectopexy. Diseases of the Colon and Rectum. 2015 Aug;**58**(8):799-807. DOI: 10.1097/DCR.0000000000000402

[45] Borie F, Coste T, Bigourdan JM, Guillon F. Incidence and surgical treatment of synthetic mesh-related infectious complications after laparoscopic ventral rectopexy. Techniques in Coloproctology. 2016 Nov;**20**(11):759-765

[46] Thauerkauf FJ, Bears OH, Hill JR. Rectal prolapse causation and surgical management. Annals of Surgery. 1970;**171**:819-835

[47] Schlinkert RT, Beart RW Jr, Wolff BG, Pemberton JH. Anterior resection for complete rectal prolapse. Diseases of the Colon and Rectum. 1985 Jun;**28**(6):409-412

[48] Frykman H, Goldberg S. The surgical management of rectal procidentia. Surgery, Gynecology & Obstetrics. 1969;**129**:1225-1230

[49] Ashari LH, Lumley JW, Stevenson AR, Stitz RW. Laparoscopically-assisted resection rectopexy for rectal prolapse: Ten years' experience. Diseases of the Colon and Rectum. 2005 May;**48**(5):982-987

[50] Tou S, Brown SR, Nelson RL. Surgery for complete (full-thickness) rectal prolapse in adults. Cochrane Database of Systematic Reviews. 2015 Nov 24;**11**:CD001758. DOI: 10.1002/14651858.CD001758.pub3

[51] Tou S, Brown SR, Malik AI, Nelson RL. Surgery for complete rectal prolapse in adults. Cochrane Database of Systematic Reviews. 2008 Oct 8;(4):CD001758. DOI: 10.1002/14651858.CD001758.pub2. Update in: Cochrane Database Syst Rev. 2015;**11**:CD001758

[52] Senapati A, Gray RG, Middleton LJ, Harding J, Hills RK, Armitage NC, Buckley L, Northover JM, PROSPER Collaborative Group. PROSPER: A randomised comparison of surgical treatments for rectal prolapse. Colorectal Disease. 2013 Jul;**15**(7):858-868. DOI: 10.1111/codi.12177

[53] Formijne Jonkers HA, Draaisma WA, Wexner SD, Broeders IA, Bemelman WA, Lindsey I, Consten EC. Evaluation and surgical treatment of rectal prolapse: an international survey. Colorectal Disease. 2013 Jan;**15**(1):115-119. DOI: 10.1111/j.1463-1318.2012.03135

[54] Dodi G, Pietroletti R, Milito G, Binda G, Pescatori M. Bleeding, incontinence, pain and constipation after STARR transanal double stapling rectotomy for obstructed defecation. Techniques in Coloproctology. 2003 Oct;**7**(3):148-153

[55] Ravo B, Amato A, Bianco V, Boccasanta P, Bottini C, Carriero A, Milito G, Dodi G, Mascagni D, Orsini S, Pietroletti R, Ripetti V, Tagariello GB. Complications after stapled hemorrhoidectomy: Can they be prevented? Techniques in Coloproctology. 2002 Sep;**6**(2):83-88

[56] Hotouras A, Ribas Y, Zakeri S, Bhan C, Wexner SD, Chan CL, Murphy JA. Systematic review of the literature on the surgical management of recurrent rectal prolapse. Colorectal Disease. 2015 Aug;**17**(8):657-664. DOI: 10.1111/codi.12946

[57] Hool GR, Hull TL, Fazio VW. Surgical treatment of recurrent complete rectal prolapse: A thirty-year experience. Diseases of the Colon and Rectum. 1997 Mar;**40**(3):270-272

[58] Pikarsky AJ, Joo JS, Wexner SD, Weiss EG, Nogueras JJ, Agachan F, Iroatulam A. Recurrent rectal prolapse: what is the next good option? Diseases of the Colon and Rectum. 2000 Sep;**43**(9):1273-1276

[59] Steele SR, Goetz LH, Minami S, Madoff RD, Mellgren AF, Parker SC. Management of recurrent rectal prolapse: Surgical approach influences outcome. Diseases of the Colon and Rectum 2006;**49**(4):440-445

[60] Cavazzoni E, Rosati E, Zavagno V, Graziosi L, Donini A. Simultaneous Delorme's procedure and inter-sphinteric prosthetic implant for the treatment of rectal prolapse and faecal incontinence: Preliminary experience and literature review. International Journal of Surgery. 2015 Feb;**14**:45-48. DOI: 10.1016/j.ijsu.2014.12.031

[61] Germain A, Perrenot C, Scherrer ML, Ayav C, Brunaud L, Ayav A, Bresler L. Long-term outcome of robotic-assisted laparoscopic rectopexy for full-thickness rectal prolapse in elderly patients. Colorectal Disease. 2014 Mar;**16**(3):198-202. DOI: 10.1111/codi.12513

Section 4

Anal Fissure and Proctitis

Chapter 5

Fissure-In-ANO

Muhammad Fahadullah and Colin Peirce

Additional information is available at the end of the chapter

http://dx.doi.org/10.5772/intechopen.76887

Abstract

This chapter provides a summary of the aetiology, diagnosis, investigation and management of anal fissure. It gives an overview of clinical anatomy and pathophysiology related to anal fissure. Focusing on anal sphincter hypertonia as the key factor for anal fissure progression, the chapter draws attention to perpetuating factors that contribute to a vicious cycle of fissure non-healing and addresses management options for these factors. This chapter also looks at the way how different treatment options for anal fissure emerged over time and uses evidence-based medicine to compare these options. "Fissure-in-ANO" concludes with summarising the treatment options and suggesting an algorithm for management of acute and chronic anal fissures.

Keywords: anal fissure, sphincter hypertonia, lateral internal sphincterotomy, glyceryl trinitrate, faecal incontinence

1. Introduction

Anal fissure, also known as fissure-in-ano, is a common cause of perianal pain. Patients often describe the pain they experience during a bowel movement as 'passing shards of glass', and the pain is often associated with rectal bleeding.

An anal fissure is an ulcer like longitudinal tear in the squamous epithelium of the anal canal, which extends from the anal verge cephalad sometimes up to the level of the dentate line. It usually causes pain both during and for 1–2 h after defecation [1]. This feature helps to distinguish anal fissure from other causes of anal pain such as perianal and ischiorectal abscesses, thrombosed haemorrhoids, viral ulcers, and others. As patients may be embarrassed about the anatomic location of their symptoms, they may present to care late in the course of their illness.

An annual incidence of 1.1 per 1000 person-years is reported, equivalent to an average lifetime risk of 7.8%. There are approximately 342,000 new cases diagnosed in the United States of America annually, a figure similar to appendectomies performed, but study estimates vary widely. One retrospective population-based study found that anal fissures most commonly affected females aged 12–24 years and males 55–64 years of age [2]. Risk factors included chronic constipation, obesity, hypothyroidism, and solid tumours.

2. Anatomy

An acute anal fissure has the appearance of a clean longitudinal tear in the anoderm, sometimes with surrounding inflammation. A chronic fissure is usually deeper and generally has exposed internal anal sphincter (IAS) fibres at its base. It is frequently associated with a hypertrophic anal papilla at its proximal aspect and with an irritated skin tag or sentinel pile at its distal aspect.

The anal canal can be described in terms of the 'surgical' and 'anatomical' anal canal. The surgical anal canal is approximately 4 cm long extending from the anal verge (anocutaneous line) to the anorectal ring (muscular ring formed at the junction of the rectum and anal canal) proximally. The anatomical anal canal is approximately 2 cm in length and extends from the anal verge distally to the dentate line (junction of the ectoderm and endoderm in the anal canal) proximally.

The epithelium of the anal canal between the anal verge below and the pectinate line above is anal mucosa. This area has somatic sensation and is the reason why anal fissures are painful. The anal canal just above the pectinate line for about 1–2 cm is called the anal transitional zone (ATZ). Above the ATZ, the anal canal is lined with columnar epithelium.

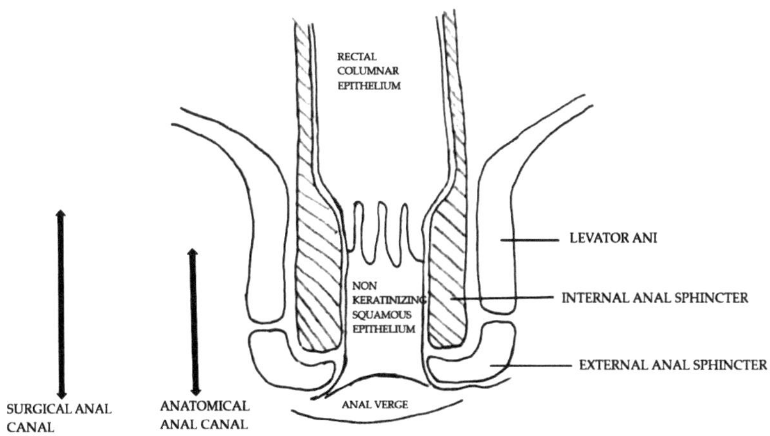

Figure 1. Schematic representation of anal canal anatomy.

http://dx.doi.org/10.5772/intechopen.76887

The inner smooth muscle layer of the colon and rectum thickens in its lowermost part over a length of 2.5–4 cm of the rectum to form the IAS. The IAS is an involuntary muscle that is in a state of continuous contraction to prevent flatal and faecal incontinence. The external anal sphincter (EAS) forms a circular tube around the anal canal. It merges proximally with the puborectalis and the levator ani muscles to form a single complex. It is supplied by the inferior rectal nerves and by a perineal branch of the fourth sacral nerve. This muscle is predominantly under voluntary contraction.

An anal fissure involves only the epithelium and when chronic in nature it involves the full thickness of the anal mucosa rendering fibres of the IAS visible. Hypertonia and hypertrophy of the IAS are commonly observed (**Figures 1–3**).

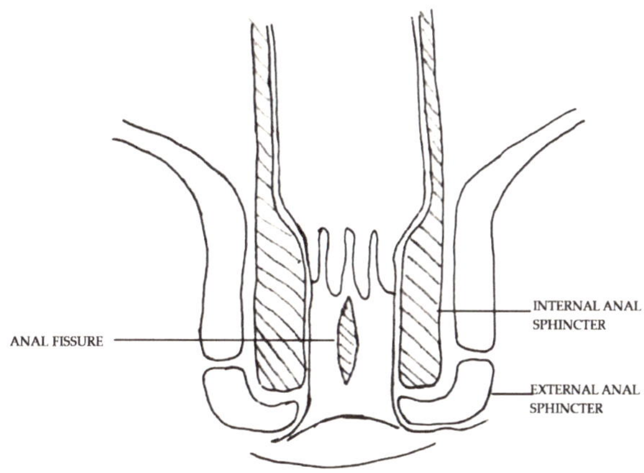

Figure 2. Schematic description of anal fissure.

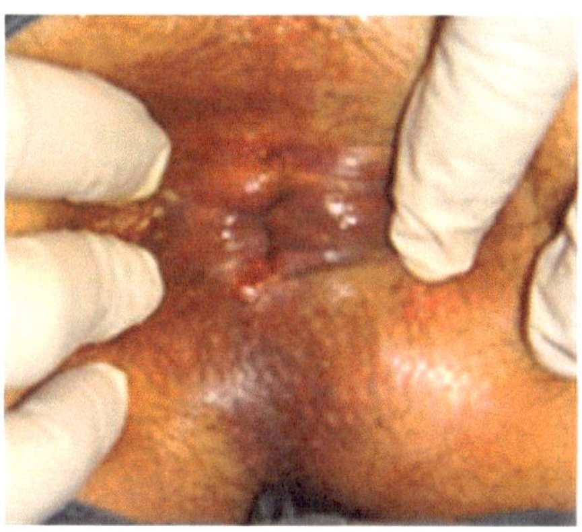

Figure 3. Posterior fissure-in-ano.

3. Pathophysiology

Different factors are involved in initiating and perpetuating the symptoms of an anal fissure. Stretching of the anal mucosa beyond its physiological limits initiates the cycle, which causes a breakdown in mucosal integrity in areas with poor muscular support i.e. an area of the relative paucity of support between the coccyx and the anorectal ring. This is followed by attempts at healing that are compromised by bowel movements that bring about repeated injury due to stretching of the whole muscular complex. The impaired healing and pain leads to persistent spasm of the IAS and an increased mean average resting luminal pressure. The persistent spasm prevents opposition of the tear leading to impaired wound healing, bacterial colonisation and progression from an acute to a chronic anal fissure in up to 40% of patients [3]. The high anal resting tone also reduces the blood supply to the posterior midline, an area of poor vascular supply of the anal canal. This explains why approximately 90% of anal fissures in both men and women are located posteriorly in the midline. Another contributing factor for posterior anal fissure is lack of clinical perineal descent in people with anal fissure which leads to repeated preferential over-stretching of the posterior anal sphincter complex and perineum. On the contrary, normally during defecation the anal sphincters and the puborectalis muscle relax, which allows the anorectal angle to widen and the perineum to descend avoiding overstretching of the posterior perineum [4].

Anterior fissures occur in 10% of patients, more commonly women and predominantly after vaginal delivery. Atypical fissures are very rare (less than 1%) and are usually found away from the midline or are multiple in number and should raise a suspicion of underlying conditions such as inflammatory bowel disease e.g. Crohn's disease, sexually transmitted diseases (human immunodeficiency disease, syphilis, or herpes), anal cancer or tuberculosis [5].

Studies have shown that people with anal fissures have increased tone [6] and hypertrophy of the IAS. The anal spasm can additionally cause ischemia of sensitive rectal tissue, which exacerbates the condition [7]. This concept is utilised in both the medical and surgical management of anal fissure.

Anal hypertonicity may aggravate perfusion to the anal canal. Studies using anorectal manometry have demonstrated hypertonia of the IAS and have shown fewer IAS relaxations in patients with chronic anal fissures [8]. Relative ischemia of the posterior anal canal has been demonstrated in chronic, non-healing anal fissures. Post-mortem studies have shown that the posterior midline of the anal canal is poorly perfused in 85% of patients. Increased IAS tone can compromise perfusion to the posterior commissure, as it increases pressure on vessels passing in a perpendicular direction through the sphincter where blood flow is already sparse [9]. Doppler laser flow studies have clearly shown lower anodermal blood flow at the fissure site compared with the posterior commissure of controls [8, 10]. Nitrous oxide synthase was also found to be intrinsically lower in individuals with fissures in one study [11].

4. Clinical findings

Patients can present with an acute or a chronic fissure-in-ano. In the acute setting, patients often complain of severe rectal pain, especially with bowel movements, described as intense

http://dx.doi.org/10.5772/intechopen.76887

and sharp and "like passing shards of glass or razor blades." The pain eases until the next bowel movement. The severity of the pain can be likened to that of urolithiasis or childbirth for some, while for others the symptoms are mild and patients need reassurance only. Patients with a chronic anal fissure complain of constant pain because of sphincter hypertrophy and spasm, with exacerbation of the pain during defecation. Passage of fresh bright red blood is less common as the initial presenting symptom. Patients are usually constipated and have a straining pattern of defecation. Painful defecation leads to avoidance of defecation and results in a vicious, self-perpetuating cycle. They tend to eat less to avoid the need for passing stool. Some patients report episodes of diarrhoea prior to the commencement of symptoms. Other patients complain of pruritus ani also, albeit this is not a common presenting symptom for a fissure. On history taking, the patient may point towards the passing of a large or hard stool as the initiating event. Anal intercourse and penetration with foreign bodies must also be enquired about, as should a personal or family history of inflammatory bowel disease.

5. Investigations

Physical examination in the left lateral position by gently separating the buttocks, and everting the anal verge usually exposes linear separation of the anoderm at the lower half of the anal canal. Severe pain can be induced with digital rectal or proctoscopic examination, so should not be attempted if a fissure is expected or demonstrable in the awake setting. If suspecting a secondary pathology and proctoscopy and digital examination are necessary, this should be done under local, regional or general anaesthesia.

If the diagnosis is unclear and the clinician is unable to see the fissure at the bedside, or a patient who is high risk for colorectal cancer and presents with significant fresh bleeding per rectum, examination under anaesthesia (EUA) with anoscopy, colonoscopy and tissue sampling may be warranted. Similarly, dependent on findings at EUA, further investigation with endoanal ultrasound, CT and MRI scanning may be required.

6. Differential diagnosis

Other conditions that can present with perianal pain and bleeding PR include thrombosed haemorrhoid, anal fistula, solitary rectal ulcer, Crohn's disease, malignancy or tuberculosis. These can be excluded by history and careful clinical assessment.

7. Classification

Anal fissures are classified on the basis of chronicity and morphological appearance. Acute fissures are defined as those with duration of symptoms of 6 weeks or less. They usually involve only the superficial mucosal layer and the base of the fissure does not have visible IAS fibres. They tend to have sharply demarcated, fresh mucosal edges, often with granulation tissue at the base [12] and often they will heal spontaneously. Lindsey et al. proposed a definition for chronic anal fissure as 'the presence of visible transverse IAS fibres at the base of an anal fissure of duration not less than 6 weeks' [13]. Over time, the IAS hypertrophies and becomes more effective in keeping the wound open and thus, prevents spontaneous wound healing. Chronic anal fissures have distinct anatomical features, such as the aforementioned visible sphincter fibres at the fissure base along with an anal papilla, sentinel pile and indurated margins.

8. Treatment options

Any treatment plan needs to address the following issues: (1) supportive measures, (2) atraumatic passage of stool, (3) pain management, (4) abnormal pattern of defecation, e.g. excessive straining, and (5) decreasing anal sphincter tone and local ischemia in patients with a hypertonic sphincter.

8.1. Supportive measures

The American Society of Colorectal Surgeons (ASCRS) recommends non-operative management as the initial treatment. ASCRS suggests that nearly 50% patients can achieve symptom resolution with the use of supportive measures such as sitz baths, bulking agents and topical anaesthetics and steroids [14–19]. A sitz bath comprises immersing the anus in lukewarm water for 10–15 min, two to three times a day. The treatment supplemented with a sitz bath regimen is associated with improved pain relief [15]. Maintenance therapy with fibre is associated with lower rates of fissure recurrence compared with placebo [18].

8.2. Atraumatic passage of stool

Constipation leads to straining and in turn usually worsening of the fissure symptoms. Laxatives, stool softeners and appropriate intake of dietary fibre are advised by ASCRS. The treatment of acute anal fissure with fibre supplementation has been associated with increased healing rates, improvement of symptoms, and prevention of recurrence [15, 18]. Fibre works by absorbing water, forming a viscus and bulky stool that promotes peristalsis and renders the stool easier to evacuate and in turn reduces the need for straining during defaecation. Stool softeners work by increasing the water content of stool and thus avoiding trauma to the anal canal lining during defecation. Mineral oil also aids to facilitate passage of stool without much stretching or abrasion of the anal mucosa, but it is not recommended for indefinite use.

8.3. Pain management

Topical anaesthetics in combination with sitz baths and the other above mentioned supporting strategies provide good pain control. Analgesics are often required for patient comfort. Non-steroidal anti-inflammatory drugs, paracetamol, and on occasion opioid analgesics are required, the latter requiring concurrent laxative use to avoid further constipation.

8.4. Abnormal pattern of defecation

Assessment of dyssynergic defaecation and anorectal feedback may be required in patients with excessive straining at defecation. A manual perineum support has been shown to help in patients with defecatory issues [20]. A novel posterior perineal device incorporated in the toilet seat has also shown improvement in pain, constipation and bleeding symptoms [21].

8.5. Decreasing sphincter tone and local ischaemia

Pharmacological and surgical options are available to manage increased IAS tone with associated local ischaemia. For chronic fissures, studies have suggested lateral internal sphincterotomy (LIS) has better results as compared to pharmacological agents [22]. ASCRS recommends LIS as the first line of treatment in the selected group of patients with no underlying faecal incontinence of any degree. The available options are discussed below.

8.5.1. Pharmacological management

Calcium channel blockers and nitrates are the most commonly used pharmacological agents. Both topical and oral forms are in use. Patients with an acute fissure can be treated with supportive measures only, but the NICE (National Institute for Health and Care Excellence) guidelines recommend using nitrates as an adjunct for 6–8 weeks followed by a re-evaluation and prescribing another course of medication if required. While for Diltiazem, NICE recommends usage only on specialist advised for those who cannot use GTN, as it's an unlicensed product. If symptoms persist then EUA and further investigation is needed.

Medical management has a much-reduced incidence of the dreaded complication of faecal incontinence but has a higher recurrence rate (around 50% for medical management as compared to 3–6% for LIS) [23–25]. This recurrence rate is similar for both calcium channel blockers and nitrates. However, patients who are already on these drugs for hypertension and ischemic heart disease may not be suitable candidates as the systemic therapy did not prevent the development of the fissure and thus may not aid in its healing.

Medical management does not provide a solution for skin tags, sentinel piles and fibrous polyps. These persist even after symptoms have resolved and can themselves cause bleeding or pain with trauma or can be a cause of faecal soilage.

8.5.1.1. Calcium channel blockers

Calcium channel blockers reduce anal tone and spontaneous activity of the sphincter by decreasing the intracellular availability of calcium. This is done by blocking the L-type calcium channels involved in the maintenance of IAS tone [26–28]. ASCRS recommends using calcium channel blockers as opposed to topical nitrates because of the superior side effect profile while having similar efficacy. In a recent systematic review and meta-analysis, topical calcium channel blockers were found to have better healing rates (21.3 vs. 38.4% unhealed fissures) as compared to oral, with fewer side effects [29].

8.5.1.1.1. Nifedipine

Studies have shown that nifedipine has a local anti-inflammatory effect [30] and produces modulating effects on the microcirculation [31]. In a trial comparing nifedipine and nitroglycerin as the treatment option, nifedipine proved to be better in healing (89 vs. 58%) and also had fewer side effects, while recurrence was frequent with both (42% with nifedipine vs. 31% with GTN) [32]. Direct comparison of oral and topical nifedipine found similar rates of healing and pain relief [27]. Given the higher incidence of systemic effects associated with oral calcium channel blockers, topical delivery is preferred.

8.5.1.1.2. Diltiazem

Recurrence is a problem for this class of drug. In one of the few long-term trials [33], more than 60% of patients experienced a recurrence within 2 years after cessation of therapy. One study reported that topical diltiazem has superior healing rates to oral diltiazem (65 vs. 38%) [34]. The main side effects include migraine and pruritus ani in 10% of patients [35, 36].

8.5.1.2. Nitrates

Myenteric nerves innervating the internal sphincter muscle of the anus produce and release nitric oxide, the chemical messenger that mediates relaxation of this muscle. Nitroglycerin, which is locally metabolised to nitric oxide, lowers the mean resting pressure of the anal sphincter when applied topically to the anus.

8.5.1.2.1. Nitroglycerin

Nitroglycerin promotes healing by decreasing pressure in the anal sphincter and concurrently increasing blood flow. For an acute fissure, NICE guidelines recommend 0.4% GTN as a second line treatment option if only supportive measures are not effective after 1 week of treatment, as a proportion of acute anal fissures heal spontaneously within 2 weeks. For chronic fissures, intra-anal application of GTN (also called glyceryl trinitrate, GTN) ointment directly to the IAS helps in fissure healing in approximately 50% [37]. Commonly used preparations come in either 0.2 or 0.4% strengths. Different doses ranging from 0.05 to 0.4% have been studied and the dose has not been shown to effect healing in three studies which compared different doses [38–40].

Headache is the main side effect occurring in at least 30% of treated patients [37]. Typically, these headaches last for no more than 30 min and occur 10–15 min after application. Hypotension is another side effect, brought about by vasodilation. It causes dizziness and thus, susceptible patients should lie down after application of the ointment to avoid dizziness. Topical GTN should be avoided within 24 h of taking erectile dysfunction medications such as Sildenafil.

A large Cochrane review compared the efficacy of 17 different therapies and concluded that topical GTN is better than placebo for anal fissures and is equivalent to botulinum toxin (BTA) injection and topical calcium channel blockers. GTN tends to cause more side effects, specifically headache [23].

8.5.1.3. Other medications and treatment options

Parasympathomimetic medications such as Bethanechol and Indoramin (alpha blocker), beta agonists like Salbutamol, natural products like Myoxinol ointment [41], egg yolks [42], and injection of sclerosing agents [43] have been tried with varying results.

Use of percutaneous posterior tibial nerve stimulation has also been suggested as a safe and effective alternative [44–46]. Studies have shown it to be some ways superior to GTN ointment for the treatment of chronic anal fissure. In a prospective randomised study of 40 patients who had persistent anal fissures despite 6 weeks of supportive measures, patients were randomised to either perianal application of GTN ointment (twice daily for 8 weeks) or percutaneous posterior tibial nerve stimulation (30–min session 2 days per week for 8 weeks). After 8 weeks of treatment, the healing rate in the percutaneous posterior tibial nerve stimulation group was 87.5 vs. 65.0% in the GTN ointment group. There were no side effects or treatment withdrawal in the nerve stimulation group as compared to 15% withdrawal in the GTN group due to headache [44].

8.5.1.4. Botulinum toxin A

The British Medical Journal (BMJ) best practice recommends using botulinum toxin (BTA) if topical agents are unsuccessful. BTA is used for performing a chemical sphincterotomy. The major effect of BTA on the IAS is blockade of sympathetic (noradrenaline mediated) neural output. This is probably a postganglionic action, involving a reduction in noradrenaline release at the neuromuscular junction causing short-term paralysis of the IAS, resulting in a reduction in anal tone [47, 48]. It can be used to treat acute and chronic anal fissures. The site of injection is still not clear and different sites have been tried (directly under the fissure or in both sides of the fissure or circumferential injections). There is no dosage or injection site with evidence of superiority. A meta-analysis shows there is no dose-dependent efficiency. The postoperative incontinence rate is not related to the dosage regardless of the type of formulation of BTA used. Also, there is no difference in healing rates with regard to the site and number of injections per session [49]. BTA has been shown to give comparable results with internal vs. external anal sphincter injection. One explanation of this is possible diffusion of the toxin from EAS to IAS [50, 51]. A second injection for an unsatisfactory response to the initial injection has shown good results where healing rates are around 60–95% after the second session of injections, with recurrence rates of 12.5% at 6 months and with no reports of anaphylaxis [23, 52, 53]. The effect is thought to last about 3 months until nerve endings regenerate allowing acute fissures (and sometimes chronic fissures) to heal and symptoms to resolve [54]. The incidence of postoperative incontinence (5–10%) [23, 49] (both faecal and flatal) needs to be considered and patients counselled regarding same.

In an updated systematic review and meta-analysis of randomised controlled trials, BTA was associated with fewer side effects than GTN but there was no difference in fissure healing or recurrence, although there was an increased incidence of transient anal incontinence [55]. Haematomas and subcutaneous infections are other commonly reported but infrequent side effects. A double-blind randomised controlled trial that compared topical diltiazem with BTA demonstrated that BTA has better healing rates in the short term but after 3 months diltiazem and BTA resulted in similar healing rates. Also, no significant difference in pain reduction was observed between the treatments [54]. ASCRS reports that BTA has similar results compared with topical therapies as first-line therapy for chronic anal fissures, and modest improvement in healing rates as second-line therapy following treatment [56].

8.5.1.5. Summation of pharmacological management

The Association of Coloproctology of Great Britain and Ireland (ACPGBI) recommends supportive treatment for both acute and chronic anal fissures, in combination with a calcium channel blocker for 6–8 weeks. If resistant to treatment, they recommend the injection of 20–25 units of BTA [57]. ASCRS recommends non-operative treatment of acute anal fissures e.g., sitz baths, psyllium fibre and bulking agents as the first step in therapy. Almost half of all patients who have an acute anal fissure will experience symptom resolution with non-operative measures [14, 15]. If symptoms persist, then pharmacological and/or surgical options should be considered.

8.5.2. Surgical options

As per a recent systematic review and meta-analysis of 148 trials, surgical intervention is significantly more effective for chronic anal fissure than medical management [24] but carries the additional potential risk of incontinence. The main contraindication to surgery for an anal fissure is impaired faecal continence, a condition that might worsen with surgery. This contraindication mostly applies to patients with minor incontinence, or who are at risk of incontinence due to a weakened sphincter complex, e.g., multiparous women and older patients. Surgery is offered to patients in whom an acute fissure is not responding to medical treatment and to those patients with chronic fissures [58–61]. No specific preoperative preparation is needed, intravenous antibiotics are not recommended [62] and preoperative enemas can be very painful for the patient and thus should be avoided.

The following are the most commonly performed operations for anal fissures.

8.5.2.1. Sphincterotomy procedures

The aim of a sphincterotomy is to release tension in the IAS by dividing it and thus allowing healing [63]. In broad terms, there are two categorised subtypes: the posterior and lateral approaches.

Posterior sphincterotomy is no longer recommended as it potentially leaves a keyhole defect [64]. Lateral internal sphincterotomy (LIS) is the gold standard surgical procedure [65]. LIS can be performed by either the open or closed technique with similar outcomes [66] and healing rates of approximately 95%. The open technique involves making an incision at the anoderm to expose the IAS and then a division of the IAS under direct vision. For the closed technique, a scalpel blade is inserted directly under the anoderm or into the intersphincteric groove and the sphincter is divided without widely incising the anal mucosa.

Common complications include recurrence in up to 6% and incontinence of flatus or stool (usually transient) in 3.4–4.4% of patients [24]. This procedure commonly involves division of the IAS from its distal end to the level of dentate line or just proximal to it. LIS has been shown to result in better quality of life than that following medical therapy. Importantly, LIS also negates any patient compliance issues associated with medical therapy. Due to this, LIS can be offered as 1st line treatment for patients with chronic anal fissures and no underlying symptoms of or predisposition to incontinence.

A modified form called a tailored sphincterotomy or fissure apex sphincterotomy involves division of the IAS up to the level of the apex of the fissure and thus it preserves more sphincteric muscle fibres. Two randomised controlled trials have reported a clinically significant reduction in incontinence with fissure apex sphincterotomy as compared the aforementioned traditional LIS [67, 68]. Another described technique is that of the calibrated sphincterotomy. A predetermined anal canal diameter (3 cm) is achieved by transecting the sphincter muscles. Results from a randomised controlled trial show equivalent healing in calibrated LIS and fissure apex LIS, but the incidence of faecal incontinence was higher in the fissure apex LIS group [69].

A recent review using three-dimensional anal ultrasonography to determine the extent of IAS division during LIS in women reported that the safest method is to divide less than 25% of the sphincter, which in women corresponds to less than 1 cm. No incontinence was observed in these patients [70]. It is important to ensure the sphincter is actually divided during LIS. A study by Farouk et al. evaluated patients with persistent fissures post-sphincterotomy with ultrasound. Almost 70% had no demonstrable division of the IAS on imaging [71]. If LIS fails, endoanal ultrasound should be performed to assess the sphincter (**Figure 4**).

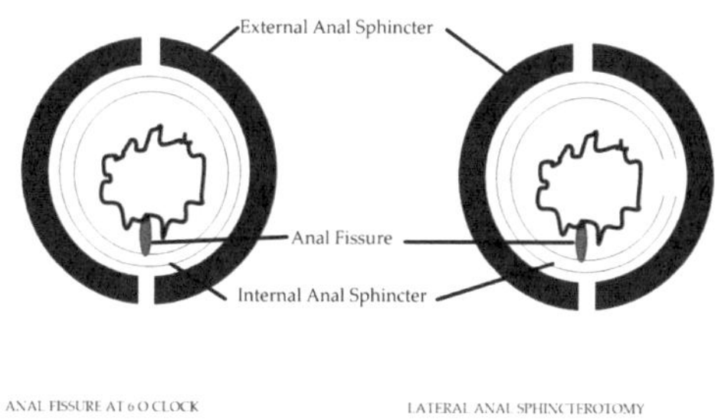

Figure 4. Diagramatic presentation of Lateral internal shincterotomy.

8.5.2.2. Anal advancement flap

This is a sphincter-saving procedure that has a very low reported incidence of postoperative minor faecal incontinence (0–6%). An anocutaneous (dermal V-Y or house) flap can be used for chronic non-healing fissures in patients with an increased risk of developing faecal incontinence (e.g. older adults, multiparous women, patients with recurrent fissures). This procedure has been shown to have good healing rates (81–100%) [53, 72]. Anal advancement flaps have been utilised as a subsequent therapy to LIS or BTA injection resulting in less postoperative pain and improved healing [73, 74].

8.5.2.3. Anal dilatation

The concept of sphincter stretching was first described by Recamier in 1838 for the treatment of proctalgia fugax and anal fissure. In 1968, Lord introduced a technique involving the insertion of four fingers of each hand into the anal canal and stretching over the course of 3–4 min. Nelson suggested abandoning the dilatation procedures by manual stretching [66]. This procedure is associated with higher rates of recurrence and incontinence [57].

A Cochrane review was performed of seven randomised controlled trials comparing anal stretch with internal sphincterotomy. The results significantly favoured sphincterotomy over anal stretch for efficacy (OR = 3.35; 95% CI = 1.55–7.26; here, OR: odds ratio, CI: confidence interval) and incontinence to flatus or faeces (OR = 4.03; 95% CI = 2.04–7.46) [23]. With the advent of endoanal ultrasound, sphincter defects after anal dilation are now readily detectable [75, 76]. In one study, IAS defects were visualised in 65% with 12.5% reporting incontinence. EAS defects were also found in 11/18 patients with incontinence [75].

Pneumatic balloon dilation (PBD) seems to be an effective, safe, easy procedure that decreases anal resting pressure without endosonographically detectable significant sphincter damage. A randomised controlled trial reported on PBD compared to LIS for the treatment of chronic anal fissure. Pneumatic dilation was performed with a 40 mm diameter, 60 mm in length anal balloon (Microvasive, Genova, Italy) with the balloon inflated to 20 psi for 6 min. Overall healing rates at 6 weeks were 83 and 92% for PBD and LIS, respectively. Based on preoperative and postoperative manometry, both techniques reduced anal pressures by ~30%. The PBD group did demonstrate mild transient faecal incontinence; however, at 24-month follow-up, the incidence of incontinence in the PBD group was 0%, but 16% in the LIS group ($p < 0.0001$) [77].

8.5.2.4. Fissurectomy

Fissurectomy entails excision of the scarred superficial skin around the anal fissure, chronic granulation tissue, hypertrophied papilla and the skin tag or sentinel pile. This then leaves a base of healthy tissue that will hopefully heal. The wound is either left open or closed primarily. In one clinical trial by Mousavi et al., fissurectomy was considered inferior to LIS. Another study by Barnes et al. reported on a combined modality of fissurectomy with BTA injection and had a 93% healing rate with only transient incontinence to flatus in 7% [78]. Fissurectomy has also been performed in conjunction with GTN or BTA injection to treat anal fissures with no recurrence and no sphincter damage on post operative endosonography [79, 80].

8.5.2.5. Surgical adjuncts

Persistence of hypertrophied papillae, skin tags and polyps often leads to patient dissatisfaction. Removal of hypertrophied anal papillae and fibrous anal polyps should be considered as a part of the surgical procedure. A randomised controlled trial found 84% of patients who had removal of the polyp, papilla or skin tag were satisfied at 2 years postoperatively as compared to only 58% of the control group [81]. A radiofrequency procedure can also useful in the eradication of these concomitant pathologies [82].

8.5.2.6. Summation of surgical management

American and British surgical societies recommend against uncontrolled manual dilatation. ASCRS recommend that LIS may be offered as first-line therapy without prior medical

http://dx.doi.org/10.5772/intechopen.76887

treatment to decrease IAS tone in a selected group of patients. The ACPGBI recommends LIS in cases of failed medical treatment, or of chronic anal fissures in association with a hypertonic anal sphincter. Modifications of the traditional sphincterotomy procedure have shown promising results. Anal advancement flaps can be an option for high-risk patients with IAS hypotonia.

8.5.3. Combination procedures

Primary wound healing can be achieved by combining anal advancement flap with LIS or BTA injection providing faster pain relief and potentially providing better functional results [83]. Theodoropoulos et al. found significantly less postoperative pain, faster healing, and fewer incontinence episodes in the tailored LIS plus flap group in comparison to the conventional LIS alone group [74]. Magdy et al. found tailored LIS with V-Y flap produced a superior healing rate, with relatively lesser complications and less rate of recurrence as compared to LIS or anal advancement flap alone [84]. In a randomised controlled trial of 99 patients, the combination of diltiazem and BTA injection was found to be as effective as LIS in patients with chronic anal fissure of the duration of 1 year or less [85].

9. Overview and comparison of side effects

Different side effects are associated with different therapies. The outcomes and side effects of the treatments for anal fissures reported in the literature are inconsistent. The recent systematic review and meta-analysis of 148 trials reported that nitrates are associated with headache in 20–30% of cases or even higher [24, 38, 86]. Higher doses do not seem to influence efficacy but do increase the side effect profile, especially headaches. Oral calcium channel blockers also have a reasonably high incidence of associated headache, but in their topical form, this is reduced to only 16%.

Variable incontinence rates have been described. LIS has been shown to have an incontinence incidence rate of 3.4–4.4%. BTA injection has a reported incontinence rate of 2.3%, GTN 1.1% and topical calcium channel blockers 1.4%. Other side effects include perianal itching and dermatitis [24]. Medical therapies have been shown to have recurrence rates as high as 50% [25].

Following chart compares different aspects of different treatment options (**Figure 5**).

	GTN	CCBs	BTA	LIS
HEALING	58%(37)	79%(29)	67.5%(1st injection)(55)	68-100%(24,25)
RECURRENCE	≈50%(24)	≈50%(24)	18.1(55)	≈6%
INCONTINENCE	1.1%(24)	1.4%(24)	2-10%(24,55)	3.4-4.4%
HEAD ACHE	20-30%	16% for topical forms	4.8%(55)	-

Figure 5. Chart comparing different aspects of different treatment options.

10. Fissures with low anal pressures

The management of anal fissure is mainly based on relieving anal hypertonicity. Patients with anterior anal fissures have been shown to have significantly lower anal pressures, suggesting a different pathophysiology in the development of these fissures [87, 88]. Low-pressure anal fissures are most commonly seen in postpartum patients. These patients are at particularly high risk for incontinence with measures directed at reducing anal hypertonia. Thus, it is especially important to approach anterior and low-pressure fissures more cautiously. It may be beneficial to perform anorectal manometry before proceeding with a treatment algorithm.

Various small studies have shown success with advancement anoplasty, or fissurectomy with advancement anoplasty, in patients with low-pressure anal fissures with reported healing rates ranging from 87 to 100% [89–91]. Advancement flap surgery may be an acceptable first approach to low-pressure fissures.

11. Novel therapies

Autologous adipose tissue injection has been shown to result in healing in 75% of treated anal fissures and 80% resolution of anal stenosis in patients with chronic anal fissure who failed previous medical and surgical therapy. Surgical treatment consisted of transplant of purified autologous fat retrieved from the hypogastrium [92]. Another reported technique is laser electrocoagulation of the fissure and its margins, leaving the IAS virtually intact. This destroys the scarred tissue and gives the tissue a chance to heal gradually from the bottom to the top of the anal ulcer of the fissure. A study reporting on 200 patients found no recurrence and no complications on follow-up [93].

A randomised prospective study compared anal self-massage with manual anal dilators and found a better resolution of an acute anal fissure in a shorter time. The anal self-massage consisted of the introduction of the patients' own index finger into the anal canal (with lubricant cream) for 10 min twice a day for the first 2 days of treatment. Following this initial 2-day strategy, patients were then instructed to perform a circular motion with the finger for 10 min twice a day for a further 5 days [94].

12. Treatment algorithm

Comparing the potential risks and benefits of different medical and surgical options as per evidence based medicine, the following treatment algorithm is proposed (**Figure 6**).

The authors favour the above algorithm, as many patients will decline the definitive treatment of surgical sphincterotomy when they are made aware of the small, but potential, complication of incontinence. Thus, commencing with supportive measures is the first step and highly unlikely to cause any lasting side effects. BTA injection is not licenced for nor present

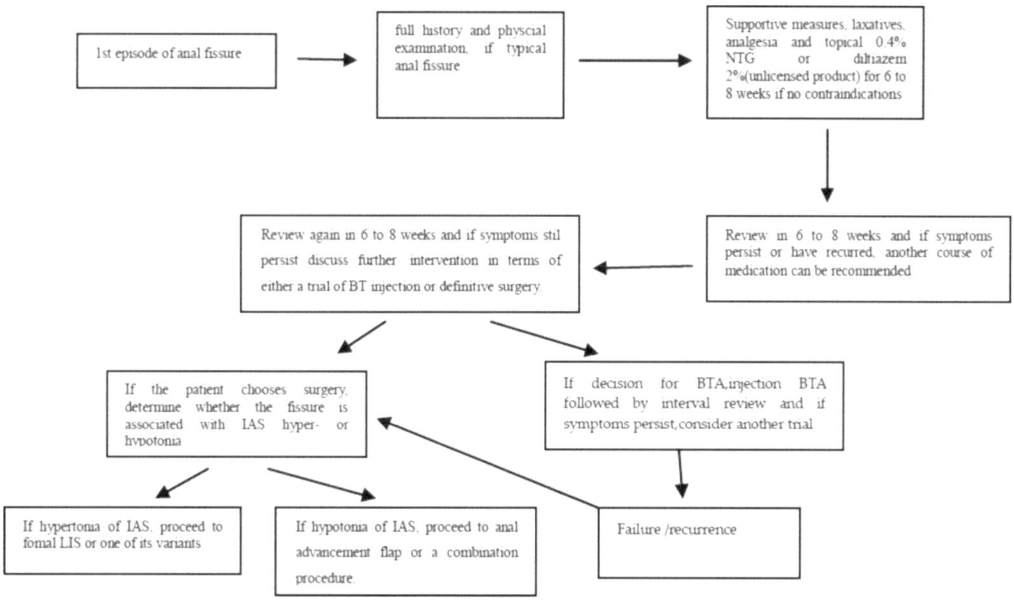

Figure 6. Algorithm for management of anal fissure.

in formal guidelines, but it is utilised by many surgeons as a bridging step between topical therapy and definitive surgery, with the added option of being able to repeat the injection if required. It often seems to be a more acceptable option to the patient also, in that it involves an injection as opposed to cutting a muscle, one sounding like a far more serious and complex operation than the other. In cases of failure of LIS, patients should be assessed with anorectal manometry and endoanal ultrasound. If the amount of sphincter divided was inadequate, repeat internal sphincterotomy can be done, or contralateral LIS can be performed [95]. Patients' wishes should be taken into consideration for further management.

13. Conclusion

An anal fissure is a painful ulceration predominantly associated with spasm of the IAS. Treatment is based on controlling pain, sphincter tone and regularisation of bowel movements. There is no consensus found among different guidelines from including Europe and America, regarding a definitive treatment algorithm with variation between health services and individual clinicians alike. While acute fissures usually heal with supportive measures and topical analgesic agents, some guidelines suggest early use of pharmacological agents even in the acute phase, while for chronic fissures medical and surgical treatments both have been recommended. Different pharmacological agents have advantages and side effects, but lateral internal sphincterotomy or its variants have been found to be best. Novel therapies have been tested but need more research. The authors like to take an aptly described 'bottom up' approach, commencing with supportive measures and topical therapies, followed by BTA injection if the patient wishes and leaving definitive surgery in the form of a sphincterotomy or advancement flap as the final treatment option.

Nomenclature

AF	Anal fissure
ASCRS	American Society of Colorectal Surgeons
LIS	Lateral internal sphincterotomy
IAS	Internal anal sphincter
ACPGBI	Association of Coloproctology of Great Britain and Ireland
BTA	Botulin toxin A
GTN	Glyceryl trinitrate
CCBs	Calcium channel blockers
PR	Per rectal
NICE	National Institute for Health and Care Excellence
RCT	Randomised control trial
PBD	Pneumatic balloon dilatation
BMJ	British Medical Journal

Author details

Muhammad Fahadullah and Colin Peirce*

*Address all correspondence to: colinpeirce@rcsi.ie

Department of Colorectal Surgery, University Hospital Limerick, Limerick, Ireland

References

[1] Goligher JC, Nixon HH, Duthie HL. Surgery of the Anus, Rectum and Colon. London: Baillière Tindall; 1980

[2] Mapel DW, Schum M, Von Worley A. The epidemiology and treatment of anal fissures in a population-based cohort. BMC Gastroenterology. 2014;**14**(1):129

[3] Madalinski MH. Identifying the best therapy for chronic anal fissure. World Journal of Gastrointestinal Pharmacology and Therapeutics. 2011;**2**(2):9-16

[4] Poh A, Tan KY, Seow-Choen F. Innovations in chronic anal fissure treatment: A systematic review. World Journal of Gastrointestinal Surgery. 2010;**2**(7):231-241

[5] Zaghiyan KN, Fleshner P. Anal fissure. Clinics in Colon and Rectal Surgery. 2011;**24**(1):22

[6] Farid M, El Nakeeb A, Youssef M, Omar W, Fouda E, Youssef T, et al. Idiopathic hypertensive anal canal: A place of internal sphincterotomy. Journal of Gastrointestinal Surgery. 2009;**13**(9):1607-1613

[7] Wray D, Ijaz S, Lidder S. Anal fissure: A review. British Journal of Hospital Medicine (London, England). 2008;**69**(8):455-458

[8] Schouten WR, Briel JW, Auwerda JJ. Relationship between anal pressure and anodermal blood flow. Diseases of the Colon and Rectum. 1994;**37**(7):664-669

[9] Klosterhalfen B, Vogel P, Rixen H, Mittermayer C. Topography of the inferior rectal artery: A possible cause of chronic, primary anal fissure. Diseases of the Colon and Rectum. 1989;**32**(1):43-52

[10] Schouten W, Briel J, Auwerda J, De Graaf E. Ischaemic nature of anal fissure. The British Journal of Surgery. 1996;**83**(1):63-65

[11] Lund JN. Nitric oxide deficiency in the internal anal sphincter of patients with chronic anal fissure. International Journal of Colorectal Disease. 2006;**21**(7):673-675

[12] Nelson RL. Anal fissure (chronic). BMJ Clin Evid 2014; 2014: 0407

[13] Lindsey I, Jones OM, Cunningham C, Mortensen NJ. Chronic anal fissure. The British Journal of Surgery. 2004;**91**(3):270-279

[14] Gough M, Lewis A. The conservative treatment of fissure-in-ano. The British Journal of Surgery. 1983;**70**(3):175-176

[15] Jensen SL. Treatment of first episodes of acute anal fissure: Prospective randomised study of lignocaine ointment versus hydrocortisone ointment or warm sitz baths plus bran. British Medical Journal (Clinical Research Ed.). 1986;**292**(6529):1167-1169

[16] Shub HA, Salvati EP, Rubin RJ. Conservative treatment of anal fissure: An unselected, retrospective and continuous study. Diseases of the Colon and Rectum. 1978;**21**(8):582-583

[17] Hananel N, Gordon PH. Re-examination of clinical manifestations and response to therapy of fissure-in-ano. Diseases of the Colon and Rectum. 1997;**40**(2):229-233

[18] Jensen S. Maintenance therapy with unprocessed bran in the prevention of acute anal fissure recurrence. Journal of the Royal Society of Medicine. 1987;**80**(5):296

[19] Gupta PJ. Randomized, controlled study comparing SITZ-bath and no-SITZ-bath treatments in patients with acute anal fissures. ANZ Journal of Surgery. 2006;**76**(8):718-721

[20] D'Hoore A, Penninckx F. Obstructed defecation. Colorectal Disease. 2003;**5**(4):280-287

[21] Tan K-Y, Seow-Choen F, Hai CH, Thye GK. Posterior perineal support as treatment for anal fissures—Preliminary results with a new toilet seat device. Techniques in Coloproctology. 2009;**13**(1):11-15

[22] Brown CJ, Dubreuil D, Santoro L, Liu M, O'Connor BI, McLeod RS. Lateral internal sphincterotomy is superior to topical nitroglycerin for healing chronic anal fissure and does not compromise long-term fecal continence: Six-year follow-up of a multicenter, randomized, controlled trial. Diseases of the Colon and Rectum. 2007;**50**(4):442-448

[23] Nelson RL, Thomas K, Morgan J, Jones A. Non surgical therapy for anal fissure. Cochrane Database of Systematic Reviews. 2012;**2**:CD003431

[24] Nelson R, Manuel D, Gumienny C, Spencer B, Patel K, Schmitt K, et al. A systematic review and meta-analysis of the treatment of anal fissure. Techniques in Coloproctology. 2017;**21**(8):605-625

[25] Ebinger SM, Hardt J, Warschkow R, Schmied BM, Herold A, Post S, et al. Operative and medical treatment of chronic anal fissures—A review and network meta-analysis of randomized controlled trials. Journal of Gastroenterology. 2017;**52**(6):663-676

[26] Cook T, Brading A, Mortensen N. Differences in contractile properties of anorectal smooth muscle and the effects of calcium channel blockade. The British Journal of Surgery. 1999;**86**(1):70-75

[27] Cook TA, Brading AF, Mortensen NJ. Effects of nifedipine on anorectal smooth muscle in vitro. Diseases of the Colon and Rectum. 1999;**42**(6):782-787

[28] Jonard P, Essamri B. Diltiazem and internal anal sphincter. The Lancet. 1987;**329**(8535):754

[29] Sahebally SM, Ahmed K, Cerneveciute R, Iqbal A, Walsh SR, Joyce MR. Oral versus topical calcium channel blockers for chronic anal fissure—A systematic review and meta-analysis of randomized controlled trials. International Journal of Surgery. 2017;**44**:87-93

[30] Fleischmann JD, Huntley HN, Shingleton WB, Wentworth DB. Clinical and immunological response to nifedipine for the treatment of interstitial cystitis. The Journal of Urology. 1991;**146**(5):1235-1239

[31] Oshiro H, Kobayashi I, Kim D, Takenaka H, Hobson RW, Durán WN. L-type calcium channel blockers modulate the microvascular hyperpermeability induced by platelet-activating factor in vivo. Journal of Vascular Surgery. 1995;**22**(6):732-741

[32] Ezri T, Susmallian S. Topical nifedipine vs. topical glyceryl trinitrate for treatment of chronic anal fissure. Diseases of the Colon and Rectum. 2003;**46**(6):805-808

[33] Nash GF, Kapoor K, Saeb-Parsy K, Kunanadam T, Dawson PM. The long-term results of diltiazem treatment for anal fissure. International Journal of Clinical Practice. 2006;**60**(11):1411-1413

[34] Jonas M, Neal KR, Abercrombie JF, Scholefield JH. A randomized trial of oral vs. topical diltiazem for chronic anal fissures. Diseases of the Colon and Rectum. 2001;**44**(8):1074-1078

[35] Bielecki K, Kolodziejczak M. A prospective randomized trial of diltiazem and glyceryltrinitrate ointment in the treatment of chronic anal fissure. Colorectal Disease. 2003;**5**(3):256-257

[36] Jonas M, Speake W, Scholefield JH. Diltiazem heals glyceryl trinitrate-resistant chronic anal fissures: A prospective study. Diseases of the Colon and Rectum. 2002;**45**(8):1091-1095

[37] Berry SM, Barish CF, Bhandari R, Clark G, Collins GV, Howell J, et al. Nitroglycerin 0.4% ointment vs placebo in the treatment of pain resulting from chronic anal fissure: A randomized, double-blind, placebo-controlled study. BMC Gastroenterology. 2013;**13**:106

[38] Carapeti E, Kamm M, McDonald P, Chadwick S, Melville D, Phillips R. Randomised controlled trial shows that glyceryl trinitrate heals anal fissures, higher doses are not more effective, and there is a high recurrence rate. Gut. 1999;**44**(5):727-730

[39] Bailey HR, Beck DE, Billingham RP, Binderow SR, Gottesman L, Hull TL, et al. A study to determine the nitroglycerin ointment dose and dosing interval that best promote the healing of chronic anal fissures. Diseases of the Colon and Rectum. 2002;**45**(9):1192-1199

[40] Scholefield J, Bock J, Marla B, Richter H, Athanasiadis S, Pröls M, et al. A dose finding study with 0.1%, 0.2%, and 0.4% glyceryl trinitrate ointment in patients with chronic anal fissures. Gut. 2003;**52**(2):264-269

[41] Martellucci J, Rossi G, Corsale I, Carrieri P, D'Elia M, Giani I. Myoxinol ointment for the treatment of acute fissure. Updates in Surgery. 2017;**69**(4):499-503

[42] Salari M, Salari R, Dadgarmoghadam M, Khadem-Rezaiyan M, Hosseini M. Efficacy of egg yolk and nitroglycerin ointment as treatments for acute anal fissures: A randomized clinical trial study. Electronic Physician. 2016;**8**(10):3035

[43] Dessily M, Charara F, Chelala E, Donfut AL, Alle JL. Injection of a sclerosing agent as first line treatment in anal fissure. Acta Chirurgica Belgica. 2014;**114**(4):261-265

[44] Ruiz-Tovar J, Llavero C. Percutaneous posterior tibial nerve stimulation vs perianal application of glyceryl trinitrate ointment in the treatment of chronic anal fissure: A randomized clinical trial. Diseases of the Colon and Rectum. 2017;**60**(1):81-86

[45] Moya P, Arroyo A, Del Mar Aguilar M, Galindo I, Giner L, Bellon M, et al. Percutaneous posterior tibial nerve stimulation in the treatment of refractory anal fissure. Techniques in Coloproctology. 2016;**20**(3):197-198

[46] Youssef T, Youssef M, Thabet W, Lotfy A, Shaat R, Abd-Elrazek E, et al. Randomized clinical trial of transcutaneous electrical posterior tibial nerve stimulation versus lateral internal sphincterotomy for treatment of chronic anal fissure. International Journal of Surgery. 2015;**22**:143-148

[47] Jankovic J, Brin MF. Therapeutic uses of botulinum toxin. The New England Journal of Medicine. 1991;**324**(17):1186-1194

[48] Jones O, Moore J, Brading A, Mortensen NMC. Botulinum toxin injection inhibits myogenic tone and sympathetic nerve function in the porcine internal anal sphincter. Colorectal Disease. 2003;**5**(6):552-557

[49] Bobkiewicz A, Francuzik W, Krokowicz L, Studniarek A, Ledwosinski W, Paszkowski J, et al. Erratum to: Botulinum toxin injection for treatment of chronic anal fissure: Is there any dose-dependent efficiency? A meta-analysis. World Journal of Surgery. 2016; **40**(12):3063

[50] Jost WH. Treatment of anal fissure with botulinum toxin A. In: Frühmorgen P, Bruch H-P, editors. Non-Neoplastic Diseases of the Anorectum: An Interdisciplinary Approach. Kluwer Academic Publishers; 2001

[51] Jost S. Chronic anal fissures treated with botulinum toxin injections: A dose-finding study with Dysport((R)). Colorectal Disease. 1999;**1**(1):26-28

[52] Wald A, Bharucha AE, Cosman BC, Whitehead WE. ACG clinical guideline: Management of benign anorectal disorders. The American Journal of Gastroenterology. 2014; **109**(8):1141-1157; (Quiz) 058

[53] Glover PH, Tang SJ, Whatley JZ, Davis ED, Jex KT, Wu R, et al. High-dose circumferential chemodenervation of the internal anal sphincter: A new treatment modality for uncomplicated chronic anal fissure: A retrospective cohort study (with video). International Journal of Surgery. 2015;**23**(Pt A):1-4

[54] Samim M, Twigt B, Stoker L, Pronk A. Topical diltiazem cream versus botulinum toxin a for the treatment of chronic anal fissure: A double-blind randomized clinical trial. Annals of Surgery. 2012;**255**(1):18-22

[55] Sahebally SM, Meshkat B, Walsh SR, Beddy D. Botulinum toxin injection vs topical nitrates for chronic anal fissure: An updated systematic review and meta-analysis of randomized controlled trials. Colorectal Disease. 2018;**20**(1):6-15

[56] Stewart DB Sr, Gaertner W, Glasgow S, Migaly J, Feingold D, Steele SR. Clinical practice guideline for the management of anal fissures. Diseases of the Colon and Rectum. 2017;**60**(1):7-14

[57] Cross KL, Massey EJ, Fowler AL, Monson JR, Acpgbi. The management of anal fissure: ACPGBI position statement. Colorectal Disease. 2008;**10**(Suppl 3):1, 7

[58] Evans J, Luck A, Hewett P. Glyceryl trinitrate vs. lateral sphincterotomy for chronic anal fissure. Diseases of the Colon and Rectum. 2001;**44**(1):93-97

[59] Libertiny G, Knight JS, Farouk R. Randomised trial of topical 0.2% glyceryl trinitrate and lateral internal sphincterotomy for the treatment of patients with chronic anal fissure: Long-term follow-up. The European Journal of Surgery. 2002;**168**(7):418-421

[60] Oettle G. Glyceryl trinitrate vs. sphincterotomy for treatment of chronic fissure-in-ano. Diseases of the Colon and Rectum. 1997;**40**(11):1318-1320

[61] Menteş BB, Irkörücü O, Akın M, Leventoğlu S, Tatlıcıoğlu E. Comparison of botulinum toxin injection and lateral internal sphincterotomy for the treatment of chronic anal fissure. Diseases of the Colon and Rectum. 2003;**46**(2):232-237

[62] Shaw D, Ternent CA. Perioperative management of the ambulatory anorectal surgery patient. Clinics in Colon and Rectal Surgery. 2016;**29**(1):7-13

[63] Rather SA, Dar TI, Malik AA, Rather AA, Khan A, Parray FQ, et al. Subcutaneous internal lateral sphincterotomy (SILS) versus nitroglycerine ointment in anal fissure: A prospective study. International Journal of Surgery. 2010;**8**(3):248-251

[64] Notaras M. Lateral Subcutaneous Sphincterotomy for Anal Fissure—A New Technique. SAGE Publications; 1969

[65] Ram E, Vishne T, Lerner I, Dreznik Z. Anal dilatation versus left lateral sphincterotomy for chronic anal fissure: A prospective randomized study. Techniques in coloproctology. Dec 3 2007:1-3

[66] Nelson RL, Chattopadhyay A, Brooks W, Platt I, Paavana T, Earl S. Operative procedures for fissure in ano. Cochrane Database of Systematic Reviews. 2011;**11**:CD002199

[67] Elsebae MM. A study of fecal incontinence in patients with chronic anal fissure: Prospective, randomized, controlled trial of the extent of internal anal sphincter division during lateral sphincterotomy. World Journal of Surgery. 2007;**31**(10):2052-2057

[68] Menteş BB, Ege B, Leventoglu S, Oguz M, Karadag A. Extent of lateral internal sphincterotomy: Up to the dentate line or up to the fissure apex? Diseases of the Colon and Rectum. 2005;**48**(2):365-370

[69] Menteş BB, Güner MK, Leventoglu S, Akyürek N. Fine-tuning of the extent of lateral internal sphincterotomy: Spasm-controlled vs. up to the fissure apex. Diseases of the Colon and Rectum. 2008;**51**(1):128-133

[70] Murad-Regadas SM, Fernandes GO, Regadas FS, Rodrigues LV, Pereira Jde J, Regadas Filho FS, et al. How much of the internal sphincter may be divided during lateral sphincterotomy for chronic anal fissure in women? Morphologic and functional evaluation after sphincterotomy. Diseases of the Colon and Rectum. 2013;**56**(5):645-651

[71] Farouk R, Monson JR, Duthie GS. Technical failure of lateral sphincterotomy for the treatment of chronic anal fissure: A study using endoanal ultrasonography. The British Journal of Surgery. 1997;**84**(1):84-85

[72] Kennedy M, Sowter S, Nguyen H, Lubowski D. Glyceryl trinitrate ointment for the treatment of chronic anal fissure. Diseases of the Colon and Rectum. 1999;**42**(8):1000-1006

[73] Patti R, Guercio G, Territo V, Aiello P, Angelo GL, Di Vita G. Advancement flap in the management of chronic anal fissure: A prospective study. Updates in Surgery. 2012;**64**(2):101-106

[74] Theodoropoulos GE, Spiropoulos V, Bramis K, Plastiras A, Zografos G. Dermal flap advancement combined with conservative sphincterotomy in the treatment of chronic anal fissure. The American Surgeon. 2015;**81**(2):133-142

[75] Nielsen MB, Rasmussen OØ, Pedersen JF, Christiansen J. Risk of sphincter damage and anal incontinence after anal dilatation for fissure-in-ano. Diseases of the Colon and Rectum. 1993;**36**(7):677-680

[76] Burnett S, Speakman C, Kamm MA, Bartram C. Confirmation of endosonographic detection of external anal sphincter defects by simultaneous electromyographic mapping. BJS. 1991;**78**(4):448-450

[77] Renzi A, Izzo D, Di Sarno G, Talento P, Torelli F, Izzo G, et al. Clinical, manometric, and ultrasonographic results of pneumatic balloon dilatation vs. lateral internal sphincterotomy for chronic anal fissure: A prospective, randomized, controlled trial. Diseases of the Colon and Rectum. 2008;**51**(1):121-127

[78] Barnes TG, Zafrani Z, Abdelrazeq AS. Fissurectomy combined with high-dose botulinum toxin is a safe and effective treatment for chronic anal fissure and a promising alternative to surgical sphincterotomy. Diseases of the Colon and Rectum. 2015;**58**(10):967-973

[79] Engel A, Eijsbouts Q, Balk A. Fissurectomy and isosorbide dinitrate for chronic fissure in ano not responding to conservative treatment. The British Journal of Surgery. 2002;**89**(1):79-83

[80] Scholz T, Hetzer F, Dindo D, Demartines N, Clavien P, Hahnloser D. Long-term follow-up after combined fissurectomy and Botox injection for chronic anal fissures. International Journal of Colorectal Disease. 2007;**22**(9):1077-1081

[81] Gupta PJ, Kalaskar S. Removal of hypertrophied anal papillae and fibrous anal polyps increases patient satisfaction after anal fissure surgery. Techniques in Coloproctology. 2003;**7**(3):155-158

[82] Filingeri V, Gravante G, Cassisa D. Clinical applications of radiofrequency in proctology: A review. European Review for Medical and Pharmacological Sciences. 2006;**10**(2):79-85

[83] Halahakoon VC, Pitt JP. Anal advancement flap and botulinum toxin A (BT) for chronic anal fissure (CAF). International Journal of Colorectal Disease. 2014;**29**(9):1175-1177

[84] Magdy A, El Nakeeb A, Fouda el Y, Youssef M, Farid M. Comparative study of conventional lateral internal sphincterotomy, V-Y anoplasty, and tailored lateral internal sphincterotomy with V-Y anoplasty in the treatment of chronic anal fissure. Journal of Gastrointestinal Surgery. 2012;**16**(10):1955-1962

[85] Gandomkar H, Zeinoddini A, Heidari R, Amoli HA. Partial lateral internal sphincterotomy versus combined botulinum toxin A injection and topical diltiazem in the treatment of chronic anal fissure: A randomized clinical trial. Diseases of the Colon and Rectum. 2015;**58**(2):228-234

[86] Perry WB, Dykes SL, Buie WD, Rafferty JF. Practice parameters for the management of anal fissures (3rd revision). Diseases of the Colon and Rectum. 2010;**53**(8):1110-1115

[87] Bove A, Balzano A, Perrotti P, Antropoli C, Lombardi G, Pucciani F. Different anal pressure profiles in patients with anal fissure. Techniques in Coloproctology. 2004;**8**(3):151-157

[88] Jenkins J, Urie A, Molloy R. Anterior anal fissures are associated with occult sphincter injury and abnormal sphincter function. Colorectal Disease. 2008;**10**(3):280-285

[89] Kenefick N, Gee A, Durdey P. Treatment of resistant anal fissure with advancement anoplasty. Colorectal Disease. 2002;**4**(6):463-466

[90] Patti R, Famà F, Barrera T, Migliore G, Di Vita G. Fissurectomy and anal advancement flap for anterior chronic anal fissure without hypertonia of the internal anal sphincter in females. Colorectal Disease. 2010;**12**(11):1127-1130

[91] Patti R, Famà F, Tornambè A, Restivo M, Di Vita G. Early results of fissurectomy and advancement flap for resistant chronic anal fissure without hypertonia of the internal anal sphincter. The American Surgeon. 2010;**76**(2):206-210

[92] Lolli P, Malleo G, Rigotti G. Treatment of chronic anal fissures and associated stenosis by autologous adipose tissue transplant: A pilot study. Diseases of the Colon and Rectum. 2010;**53**(4):460-466

[93] Pappas AF, Christodoulou DK. A novel minimally invasive treatment for anal fissure. Annals of Gastroenterology. 2017;**30**(5):583

[94] Gaj F, Biviano I, Candeloro L, Andreuccetti J. Anal self-massage in the treatment of acute anal fissure: A randomized prospective study. Annals of Gastroenterology. 2017;**30**(4):438-441

[95] Liang J, Church JM. Lateral internal sphincterotomy for surgically recurrent chronic anal fissure. The American Journal of Surgery. 2015;**210**(4):715-719

Chapter 6

Radiation Proctitis

Radzislaw Trzcinski, Michal Mik, Lukasz Dziki and Adam Dziki

Additional information is available at the end of the chapter

http://dx.doi.org/10.5772/intechopen.76200

Abstract

Pelvic radiotherapy (RT) has become a vital component of curative treatment for various pelvic malignancies. The fixed anatomical position of the rectum in the pelvis and the close proximity to the prostate, cervix, and uterus, makes the rectum especially vulnerable to secondary radiation injury resulting in chronic radiation proctitis (CRP). Clinical symptoms associated with CRP are commonly classified by the EORTC/RTOG late radiation morbidity scoring system. Rectal bleeding is the most frequent symptom of CRP occurring in 29–89.6% of patients. Endoscopy is essential to determine the extent and severity of CRP as well as to exclude other possible causes of inflammation or malignant disease. Typical endoscopic findings of rectal mucosal damage in the course of radiation-induced proctitis include friable mucosa, rectal mucosal hypervascularity, and telangiectases. There is no consensus available for the treatment of CRP, and different modalities present a recurrence rate varying from 10 to 30%. CRP can be managed conservatively, and also includes ablation (formalin enemas, radiofrequency ablation, YAG laser or argon plasma coagulation) as well as some patients require surgery. Although modifications of radiation techniques and doses are continually being studied to decrease the incidence of CRP, trials investigating preventive methods have been disappointing to date.

Keywords: pelvic malignancies, radiotherapy, radiation proctitis

1. Introduction

The discovery of X-rays in 1895 by Wilhelm Röntgen was followed 2 years later by the discovery by Walsh of the damaging effects of X-irradiation on the gastrointestinal tract. In 1912, Regaud et al. described delayed changes in the small intestine of a dog following irradiation. Krause and Ziegler believed that harmful effects of X-irradiation on the small intestine were caused by the proliferation of intestinal bacteria [1–4]. In 1917, the first clinical report of a patient who developed severe intestinal injury following the use of radiation therapy for treatment of malignant disease was published [4]. Then, in 1930, Buie gave the first description of factitial proctitis, which referred to chronic radiation-induced injury to the rectum in a group of patients who had undergone pelvic irradiation [3, 5].

Radiotherapy (RT) has now become a common treatment for many cancers involving the pelvis, with around 12,000 patients undergoing pelvic radiotherapy in the UK each year, over 100,000 American patients annually receiving therapeutic pelvic radiation and up to 300,000 patients per year worldwide [2, 6, 7]. Pelvic radiotherapy is a vital component of curative treatment typically used in urological, gynecological and gastrointestinal tract cancers (prostate, urinary bladder, cervical, uterine, rectal and anal malignancies). Pelvic radiation is administered either as neoadjuvant or adjuvant therapy. After pelvic irradiation, the rectum is the commonest site of injury within the gastrointestinal tract. The fixed anatomical position of the rectum in the pelvis and the close proximity to the prostate, cervix and uterus make the rectum especially vulnerable to secondary radiation injury resulting in proctitis [8–16].

The anterior rectal wall is in close proximity to and partly in continuity with the therapeutic target organs (prostate, uterus) [17, 18]. Although the development of late gastrointestinal toxicity following pelvic radiotherapy is not entirely dose related, there is a rapid rise in the number of rectal complications when the cumulative mean rectal dose and the cumulative maximum dose exceed 75 Gy, and there is also evidence that the incidence of severe complications rises sharply above a total dose of 80 Gy [19–21]. Treatment for prostate carcinoma typically receives 75 Gy over 7 to 8 weeks, and cervical carcinoma might receive 45 Gy of the typical external beam radiotherapy (EBRT) plus a variable dosing of brachytherapy [22]. There is an increasing risk of rectal toxicity ranging from 2% for patients receiving ≤50 Gy to 15–18% for patients receiving ≥80 Gy [20].

Acute radiation proctitis is encountered by up to 75% of patients receiving conventional pelvic radiotherapy and is defined as an inflammatory process involving only the superficial mucosa. It occurs within 1–6 weeks of radiation treatment and is generally self-limited with symptom resolution often within 3 months after the onset of therapy [2, 4, 6, 8, 12, 23–25]. There is some evidence to suggest that moderate or severe chronic radiation proctitis is at least twice more likely to occur in those initially experiencing severe acute proctitis [22, 26]. Chronic radiation proctitis occurs months to years after treatment with a large majority within 2 years post radiotherapy, and this entity is a troublesome complication in those undergoing pelvic irradiation for any cause. The incidence of late complications is about 2.5–30%; although with improving techniques and newer modalities of radiation therapy and minimizing the dose of radiation to the rectum, the incidence is decreasing [2, 4, 6, 8, 12, 15, 20, 22–24, 27–31].

The development of postradiation rectal toxicity is not entirely dose, volume and fractionation schedule related. It also depends on a complex interaction of physical, patient-related and genetic factors, but these have been poorly characterized to date [7]. Many patients suffer progressive disease that may be life-long. There are a number of predisposing factors that may play a role in the increased risk of developing chronic radiation proctitis: age > 60 years, low BMI, diabetes, cardiovascular disease, hypertension, peripheral vascular disease, use of anticoagulants, inflammatory bowel disease, hormonal therapy, collagen vascular disease, atherosclerosis, preexisting inflammatory bowel disease, smoking, pelvic inflammatory conditions, previous abdominopelvic surgery and possibly secondary anatomical changes with intraabdominal adhesions leading to immobility of intestinal loops in the radiation field (e.g., hysterectomy), radiation dosages to the lower pelvis >54 Gy, the volume of rectum irradiated, RT technique and dose per fraction, previous concomitant or subsequent chemotherapy, ataxia-telangiectasia gene and HIV infection [2, 4, 6, 8, 12, 16, 20, 22, 24, 32, 33].

2. Pathology

Any part of the gastrointestinal tract may be affected by the radiation [4]. Radiotherapy induces long-term changes in bowel function as a result of progressive endothelial dysfunction, which includes ischemia and subsequent fibrosis. The same processes may cause dysfunction in other pelvic organs; therefore, Andreyev et al. defined this disorder as "pelvic radiation disease" (PRD). "Proctitis" suggests that there is an ongoing inflammation, whereas there is inflammation during and immediately after radiotherapy, but, by 3 months or more, inflammation has been replaced almost entirely by progressive ischemia and fibrosis. PRD currently affects as many each year as develop inflammatory bowel disease (IBD) has a spectrum of symptoms identical to IBD and shares some of its pathological features. Unlike IBD, however, we know that PRD starts with the initiation of radiotherapy. During therapeutic irradiation of a pelvic malignancy, parts of distal small bowel, caecum, transverse and sigmoid colon and rectum are often also irradiated. Additionally, the pancreas and proximal small bowel may also receive some irradiation if para-aortic nodes are treated. Moreover, in the chronic phase of the disease, there is minimal inflammation; "-itis" signifies inflammation, and so describing the situation as "-itis" is misleading. So, Andreyev et al. suggest the term "radiation proctopathy" to be better. This is not further discussed here because they go beyond the scope of this chapter which focuses mainly on chronic radiation proctitis [27, 34–36].

3. Clinical features

Radiation-induced bowel toxicity has been dominated by the application of scoring scales that are based on clinical symptoms [7, 27]. Intensity of chronic radiation proctitis is also scored with regard to clinical symptoms. Numerous grading systems are used in the literature to assess rectal toxicity following radiotherapy. Currently, clinical symptoms associated with CRP are most commonly classified by the EORTC/RTOG late radiation morbidity scoring system (the European Organization for Research and Treatment of Cancer/Radiation Therapy Oncology Group score for late rectal toxicity) (**Table 1**) [3, 7, 22, 26, 28, 34, 37–40].

Chronic radiation proctitis may be associated with diarrhea, tenesmus, mucus discharge, ulcers and abdominal/rectal pain, but bleeding is the most common symptom with potential iron deficiency anemia that may require hospitalization and even blood transfusions. Refractory bleeding is a real challenge to clinicians. The frequency of rectal bleeding after RT

Proctitis grades	Radiation-induced clinical symptoms
0	None
1	Mild diarrhea, mild cramping, bowel movements up to five times daily, slight rectal discharge or bleeding, mild anal pain and mild rectal tenesmus
2	Moderate diarrhea and colic, bowel movements more >5 times daily, excessive rectal mucus or intermittent rectal bleeding
3	Obstruction or persistent bleeding requiring surgery
4	Necrosis/perforation/fistula
5	Fatal toxicity (sepsis, multiple organ dysfunction syndrome)

Table 1. The EORTC/RTOG scoring system (Radiation Therapy Oncology Group/European Organization for Research and Treatment of Cancer score for late radiation proctitis).

is said to occur in 29–89.6% of patients, and it is the second most common reason for referral to a gastroenterologists after radiotherapy. Some degree of abdominal or rectal pain affects up to 30% of all patients after radiotherapy, and it influences daily living in about 10%. Patients may present symptoms of obstructed defecation because of strictures accompanied with constipation, rectal pain, urgency and sometimes fecal incontinence. Fistulas into adjacent organs (e.g., vagina) may also occur[4, 6–8, 10, 12, 16, 23, 25, 29, 31, 35, 40, 41].

Because of the nature of radiation injury, the incidence of severe complications (transfusion-dependent bleeding, fistula formation, rectal stricture and bowel obstruction, perforation, secondary malignancy) increases with time. Estimates of the significance of these severe consequences of radiotherapy have varied between 0.5 and 30%, but more reasonable estimates suggest that these occur between 15 and 20% over 20–30 years [4, 7, 12, 42]. Late injury to the rectum usually occurs in the first 2–3 years after treatment and the incidence then plateaus [25, 43].

4. Endoscopic findings

Each patient who has undergone radiotherapy for pelvic malignancies and reports symptoms suggestive of radiation-induced proctitis should be suspected of this entity, even if irradiation was performed many years ago. Endoscopy, in any case, is important to determine the extent and severity of chronic radiation proctopathy as well as to exclude other possible causes of inflammation or malignant disease [8]. Abnormal endoscopic findings after pelvic radiotherapy include congested mucosa, telangiectasia, erythema or pallor, ulceration, stricture, fistula and necrosis. Fragile rectal mucosa is prone to bleeding. Telangiectasia of the rectal mucosa which are very frequent and a major cause of bleeding may resolve spontaneously after 3 years. However, the prevalence of telangiectases in unselected patients is unknown [8, 18, 29, 31, 32, 43].

Endoscopic evaluation of acute radiation proctitis shows edematous, dusky red rectal mucosa, whereas endoscopy of chronic radiation proctitis shows mucosal atrophy, ectatic superficial capillaries, tortuous blood vessels, telangiectasias, variable stenosis, strictures and fistulas [6]. Characteristic endoscopic changes of rectal mucosal damage in the course of radiation proctitis are shown in **Figure 1**.

http://dx.doi.org/10.5772/intechopen.76200

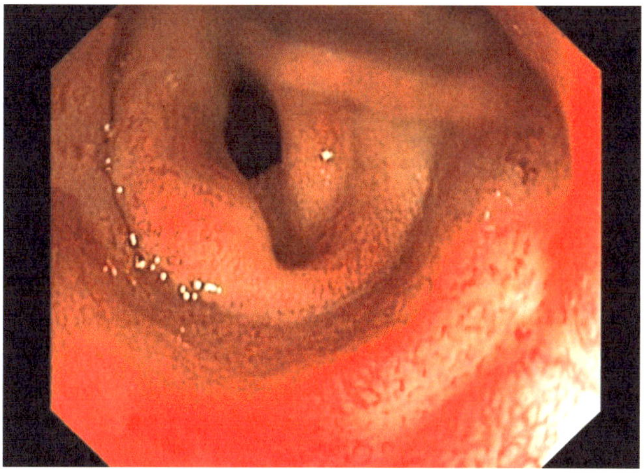

Figure 1. Typical endoscopic appearance of rectal mucosal damage in the course of radiation proctitis—congested and friable mucosa, extensive rectal mucosal hypervascularity, tortuous blood vessels and telangiectases.

It is also important to highlight that due to the possibility of initiating chronic, poorly healing wounds and the risk of possible complications of sepsis, fistula formation and also the increased risk of bleeding, biopsy of devitalized rectal tissues should be avoided as they do not contribute to the diagnosis of chronic radiation proctopathy. Rectal biopsy is only justified if any malignancy is suspected or in a case of important therapeutic consequences [8, 12, 44].

5. Differential diagnosis

Radiation-induced proctitis should be suspected in any patient after pelvic radiotherapy who presents the symptoms of this entity. Acute radiation proctitis may mimic allergic or eosinophilic colitis, but the history will allow accurate diagnosis. However, endoscopy is essential to exclude other causes of acute or chronic proctitis such as infectious colitis, inflammatory bowel disease, diversion colitis, ischemic colitis, angiodysplasia, diverticular colitis and concomitant other malignancies [6, 8].

6. Treatment: medical and surgical

Radiation-induced proctopathy is unlikely to find one treatment modality that works for all patients. Acute radiation-induced proctitis is managed conservatively and includes hydration, antidiarrheals and steroid or 5-aminosalicylate enemas [12].

There is no consensus available for the treatment of chronic radiation proctopathy, and the different modalities present a recurrence rate varying from 10 to 30%. Chronic radiation-induced proctitis can be managed conservatively (anti-inflammatory agents, sucralfate, short-chain fatty acids, hyperbaric oxygen therapy, antioxidants) and also includes ablation (formalin enemas, radiofrequency ablation, YAG laser or argon plasma coagulation) and surgery [12]. There was also a case report of successful treatment of a patient with severe refractory hemorrhagic radiation proctitis with low dose of oral thalidomide [6, 45]. It is very important to realize, when considering invasive treatment that chronic radiation-induced proctitis can improve over time without any treatment [8].

6.1. 5-Aminosalicytic acid (5-ASA)

The mechanism of anti-inflammatory action of 5-ASA is the inhibition of prostaglandin synthesis. 5-ASA may also inhibit folate-dependent enzymes and free radical-scavenging activity [12].

6.2. Steroids

Steroids (prednisone, betamethasone, hydrocortisone) have multiple mechanisms of action that produce anti-inflammatory effects which extend from stabilization of lysosomes in neutrophils to prevent degranulation to upregulation of anti-inflammatory genes via binding to glucocorticoid receptors [12]. Steroids have been used to treat radiation proctitis both alone and in combination with other agents [28]. The addition of *metronidazole* to oral mesalazine and betamethasone enemas was associated with a reduction in rectal bleeding, diarrhea and ulcers [8].

6.3. Sucralfate and pentosan polysulfate (PPS)

Sucralfate (2–3 g of sucralfate in a 15–20 ml suspension, oral sucralfate, paste) adheres to mucosal cells and stimulates epithelial healing and the formation of protective epithelial barrier while PPS (a synthetic derivative of a glycosaminoglycan) is thought to reduce epithelial permeability and prevent adherence similar to sucralfate. Moreover, sucralfate has been found to induce a better clinical response than anti-inflammatories in patients with CRP. Based on a Cochrane review, sucralfate enemas were more effective than corticosteroid or mesalazine enemas [8, 12, 22, 28, 35, 39]. A novel method of rectal administration of sucralfate via a low-volume sucralfate paste (two sucralfate 1 g tablets mixed with 4.5 ml of water) was reported by McElvanna et al. Clinical improvement was reported in 73% of patients, and 32% had resolution of all symptoms [39].

PPS, a fibrinolytic, anti-inflammatory and mucoprotective agent, resolved symptoms in nine of thirteen patients with established chronic radiation proctitis [20].

6.4. Short-chain fatty acids (SCFAs)

Short-chain fatty acids are the main energy source for colonocytes and stimulate colonic mucosal proliferation. The most important product of SCFA is butyric acid. They also exert a vasodilatatory effect on the arteriole walls to improve blood flow. SCFAs were found to accelerate the healing process, with a significant early reduction in bleeding episodes and endoscopic scores. One of two small randomized, placebo-controlled trials noted more rapid improvement in symptoms and endoscopic findings in a group of patients using a butyrate-containing SCFAs solution over a 5-week period compared with placebo controls [12, 22, 28].

6.5. Formalin

Formalin application has been demonstrated to be generally effective and safe in hemorrhagic proctitis and, however, may cause complications such as chronic anorectal pain, fever, fecal incontinence, rectosigmoid necrosis with or without perforation, enteric fistula formation, anal and rectal strictures as well as pelvic sepsis. Topical formalin instillation (4% solution, formalin-soaked pads with up to 10% solution) may be repeated in case of recurrent bleeding and combined with other methods [9, 12, 20, 31, 35, 40, 41, 46, 47]. Formalin enemas probably reduce mucosal blood flow, sclerose and seal fragile telangiectasias through chemical cauterization to prevent further bleeding with reported success rate of 48–100%. Direct contact with formalin for 2–3 minutes (via formalin solution installation through endoscope or Foley catheter or soaked gauze) causes chemical cauterization of neovasculature [9, 12, 35, 40, 41, 47].

6.6. Antioxidants

As oxidative stress is thought to be an important factor in the development of chronic radiation proctitis, antioxidants have been used in an attempt to limit tissue damage. The use of vitamins E (400 IU three times daily), C (500 mg three times daily) and A (10,000 IU twice daily for 90 days) significantly reduced proctitis symptoms (diarrhea, bleeding, urgency) [8, 12, 48].

6.7. Endoscopic treatment

A variety of endoscopic coagulation devices (e.g., Nd:YAG laser, argon plasma coagulation, bipolar electrocoagulation, and heater probe) deliver thermal coagulation to the focal bleeding telangiectasia and should be reserved for patients suffering from significant hemorrhagic proctitis. There have been also reports on endoscopic balloon dilatation and stenting for radiation-induced rectal strictures [12, 28].

Argon plasma coagulation (APC)—monopolar diathermy is used to ionize the argon gas which coagulates the telangiectatic vessels in a noncontact fashion (0.8–3.0 mm from the target). Many gastroenterologists consider APC as the treatment of choice for CRP. A complete resolution of bleeding is obtained in 70–80% of patients, but an average of three treatment sessions is required. On the other hand, we have to realize severe complications that may happen after this procedure which is performed in chronically ischemic tissues (deep ulceration, fistulation, rectal stenosis, rebound bleeding, long-term pain, perforation, rectovaginal fistula and even bowel explosions in inadequately prepared bowels). The development of rectal ulcers after APC is thought to be a consequence of thermal injury. On the basis of anecdotal evidence, APC is commonly ineffective in patients with very heavy bleeding [8, 12, 15, 20, 25, 31, 35, 47, 49].

YAG laser coagulation has a similar benefit as APC with a limited depth of penetration and the possibility for precise application. The major risk for laser coagulation is transmural necrosis, with perforation or stricture formation. Nevertheless, the laser is expensive and not widely available [8, 12, 20, 31].

Trans-anal rectoscopic ball diathermy (TARD)—monopolar diathermy coagulation is used to coagulate radiation-induced hemorrhagic telangiectasia (RIHT). Treatment involves applications of monopolar diathermy to the rectal mucosa over the affected areas, targeting the central "feeding vessel" of the telangiectatic spots. TARD is a safe and effective modality with 85% of patients reporting immediate symptomatic control with no significant morbidity [46].

Endoscopic cryoablation (cryospray ablation therapy) involves noncontact application of liquid nitrogen or carbon dioxide gas to the tissue and offers superficial ablation of mucosa in patients with CRP. Cryotherapy has been suggested as a safe and effective method for bleeding in CRP. Hou et al. reported a series of ten patients with hemorrhagic radiation proctitis treated with endoscopic cryoablation. Overall subjective clinical scores improved as determined by the Radiation Proctitis Severity Assessment Scale from 27.7 to 13.6 ($p = 0.003$), and symptom improvement correlated with endoscopic improvement. Cryotherapy is novel and up to date, and there is very limited data [15, 24, 47].

6.8. Hyperbaric oxygen therapy (HBOT)

HBOT involves patients breathing pure oxygen in a pressurized room or tube. Under these conditions, the lungs can gather more oxygen than at normal air pressure. Higher oxygenated blood may inhibit bacterial growth and stimulate the release of growth factors and stem cells; thus, it affects and promotes wound healing. Increased oxygen pressure to telangiectatic vessels reverses the ischemic component of chronic radiation proctopathy and promotes angiogenesis with healing of rectal mucosa. Two randomized controlled trials (RCTs) and one nonrandomized comparative study examined HBOT for treatment of radiation proctitis. First, RTC showed a significantly greater proportion of HBOT patients demonstrating at least moderate healing of proctitis in comparison with sham treatment group immediately after completion of treatment (87.5 vs. 62.5%, $p = 0.0009$). The second RTC reported that treatment with HBOT significantly decreased the prevalence of radiation proctitis compared to symptomatic treatment alone at 6-month follow-up (76.9 vs. 42.9%, $p = 0.026$). The nonrandomized comparative study found that HBOT patients required statistically more blood transfusions than APC (argon plasma coagulation) patients at 1-month ($p = 0.03$) and 2-month follow-up ($p = 0.04$). This difference was nonsignificant after 3 months. Side effects after HBOT may include barotrauma (ear pain), myopia and confinement anxiety [8, 24, 31, 47, 50].

As late radiation injury is characterized by abnormal angiogenesis, the future will show whether it will be possible to develop drugs to treat radiation proctitis with angiogenic factors as their target. Inhibitors of angiogenic factors such as angiogenin and fibroblast growth factor 1 (FGF1) might be also effective for treating CRP [51].

6.9. Surgery

Surgery is a feasible curative option for severe cases refractory to medical treatment; however, there is no universally agreed surgical first-line approach in the literature, indicating which patients should undergo surgery nor which surgical procedure is optimal. On the other hand, surgery in previously irradiated patients is often extremely difficult because of fibrosis within the abdomen and carries significantly higher risks of complications and mortality than surgery in nonirradiated patients. Thus, surgery is reserved solely as a last resort; nevertheless, the challenge for clinicians is to develop an evidence-based consensus to decide when

http://dx.doi.org/10.5772/intechopen.76200

Indications for surgery
• Failure of conservative treatment (intractable bleeding)
• Strictures and rectal obstruction
• Rectal or rectosigmoid perforation
• Fistulas (e.g., recto-vaginal, rectovesical, recto-urethral)
• Uncontrollable rectal pain

Table 2. Indications for surgery in patients with chronic radiation proctitis.

the benefits of surgery outweigh the risks in the group of patients refractory to conservative treatment [7, 8, 14, 23, 28, 41]. Reported data on the increasing risk over time of complications requiring operative intervention show that 4–10% of patients are affected over 5–10 years and up to 20% over 20 years [27]. Generally, approximately 2.6–10% and even up to one-third of the patients will undergo surgery due to complications of radiation proctitis. The preferred surgical approach is not universally agreed. Surgery for CRP mainly involves either diverting loop colostomy or resection without primary anastomosis. The issue with diversion alone for CRP is that it does not remove the damaged tissue, and leaving it in situ leaves the patient at risk of further bleeding, perforation, obstruction and abscess formation. Therefore, some authors advocate that if patients are fit enough, resection should be the first-line therapy, and defunctioning stoma reserved for patients who are poor surgical candidates for resection. Another option is resection with loop ileostomy. Diversion of stool or the urinary stream with an ostomy or a suprapubic catheter should be considered in almost all cases where repair is attempted. In cases of complicated fistulous disease, particularly when accompanied by significant pain and incontinence, a proctectomy or pelvic exenteration with or without reconstruction is recommended. In cases of severe and intractable bleeding, proctectomy may be the only option [8, 12, 20, 23, 41]. The most common indications for surgical management in patients with chronic radiation proctitis are shown in **Table 2** [12, 20, 23, 28].

When surgical treatment is needed, most studies demonstrate poor outcomes with complication rates of 15–80% (sepsis, wound dehiscence, bowel obstruction, de novo rectal fistula) and a mortality of 3–9% and even up to 25% [8, 12, 20]. In contrary to diversion alone, major resectional surgery carries higher morbidity and mortality risks. Mortality and morbidity vary from 0 to 44% and from 0 to 11% for diversion only vs. 0–100% and 0–14% in cases of resectional surgery [23].

7. Prevention

Although modifications of radiation techniques and doses are continually being studied to decrease the incidence of radiation-induced proctitis, trials investigating preventive methods have been disappointing to date. The role of pharmacological and nutritional therapy in reducing radiation-induced gut disease has been evaluated in a variety of experimental settings, including animal models (e.g., pravastatin, teduglutide). Agents that reverse fibrosis might be useful but need to be taken for many months to produce benefit. Many treatments have potential antifibrotic activity (liposomal copper-zinc superoxide dismutase, pentoxifylline with or without high-dose vitamin E and hyperbaric oxygen). Balsalazide used 5 days before and up to 2 weeks after pelvic radiotherapy proved an improvement in toxicity grades, particularly pertaining to proctitis. Diets enriched with glutamine, arginine and vitamin E have been shown to have a protective effect on the intestinal mucosa of rats treated with radiotherapy. However, there are no trials assessing the role of dietary supplements in attenuating the development of chronic radiation enteritis in humans [2, 7, 12, 35, 48]. Preventative measures (e.g., the use of rectal misoprostol, oral or rectal sucralfate) have not made a significant contribution to decrease the incidence of radiation proctitis. However, data available in the literature are ambiguous. Khan et al. found that misoprostol rectal suppositories given prior to each radiotherapy session reduced acute and chronic proctitis syndrome [12, 22].

Optimizing the radiotherapy planning by using planning constraints reduces the irradiated rectal volume and, thus, decreases the risk of rectal toxicity. Appropriate packing to push the rectum and bladder away from the radioactive source helps in reducing the incidence of radiation proctitis. There is also evidence in favor of genetic variants in the development of radiation toxicity. Therefore, there is a role for further studies to identify high-risk patients based on genetic biomarkers [4, 8].

Author details

Radzislaw Trzcinski*, Michal Mik, Lukasz Dziki and Adam Dziki

*Address all correspondence to: trzcinskir@wp.pl

Department of General and Colorectal Surgery, Medical University of Lodz, Lodz, Poland

References

[1] Somozy Z, Horváth G, Telbisz Á, et al. Morphological aspects of ionizing radiation response of small intestine. Micron. 2002;**33**:167-178

[2] Theis VS, Sripadam R, Ramani V, et al. Chronic radiation proctitis. Clinical Oncology. 2010;**22**:70-83

[3] Bielecki K. Chronic radiation proctitis (CRP). Nowa Medycyna. 2014;**3**:99-106

[4] Sharma B, Pandey D, Chauhan V, et al. Radiation proctitis. JIACM. 2005;**6**(2):146-151

[5] Buie LA, Malmgren GE. Factitial proctitis. Transactions American Proctologic Society. 1930;**29**:80-84

[6] Weisenberg E. Anus and Perianal Area – Radiation Proctitis. Last major update October 2014. Available from: http://www.pathologyoutlines.com/topic/anusradiationproctitis.html

[7] Andreyev HJN. Gastrointestinal problems after pelvic radiotherapy: The past, the present and the future. Clinical Oncology. 2007;**19**:790-799

[8] Vanneste BGL, De Voorde LV, de Ridder RJ, et al. Chronic radiation proctitis: Tricks to prevent and treat. International Journal of Colorectal Disease. 2015;**30**:1293-1303

[9] Dziki Ł, Kujawski R, Mik M, et al. Formalin therapy for hemorrhagic radiation proctitis. Pharmacological Reports. 2015;**67**:896-900

[10] Williams HRT, Vlavianos P, Blake P, et al. The significance of rectal bleeding after pelvic radiotherapy. Alimentary Pharmacology & Therapeutics. 2005;**21**:1085-1090

[11] Denton AS, Andreyev HJN, Forbes A, Maher EJ. Systematic review for non-surgical intervention for the management of late radiation proctitis. British Journal of Cancer. 2002;**87**(2):134-143

[12] Do NL, Nagle D, Poylin VY. Radiation proctitis: Current strategies in management. Gastroenterology Research and Practice 2011;**2011**:9. Article ID 917941. DOI: 10.1155/2011/917941

[13] Varma JS, Smith AN, Busuttil A. Function of the anal sphincters after chronic radiation injury. Gut. 1986;**27**:528-533

[14] Counter SF, Froese DP, Hart MJ. Prospective evaluation of formalin therapy for radiation proctitis. American Journal of Surgery. 1999;**177**:396-398

[15] Tang SJ, Bhaijee F. Chronic radiation proctopathy and colopathy. Video Journal and Encyclopedia of GI Endoscopy. 2013;**1**:307-308

[16] Babb RR. Radiation proctitis: A review. The American Journal of Gastroenterology. 1996; **91**:1309-1311

[17] Hovdenak N, Fajardo LF, Hauer-Jensen M. Acute radiation proctitis: A sequential clinicopathologic study during pelvic radiotherapy. International Journal of Radiation Oncology, Biology, Physics. 2000;**48**:1111-1117

[18] Krol R, Smeenk RJ, van Lin ENJT, et al. Systematic review: Anal and rectal changes after radiotherapy for prostate cancer. International Journal of Colorectal Disease. 2014; **29**:273-283

[19] Gami B, Harringtom K, Blake P, et al. How patients manage gastrointestinal symptoms after pelvic radiotherapy. Alimentary Pharmacology & Therapeutics. 2003;**18**:987-994

[20] O'Brien PC. Radiation injury of the rectum. Radiotherapy and Oncology. 2001;**60**:1-14

[21] Ogino I, Kitamura T, Okamoto N, et al. Late rectal complications following high dose rate intracavitary brachytherapy in cancer of the cervix. International Journal of Radiation Oncology, Biology, Physics. 1995;**31**:725-734

[22] Kennedy GD, Heise CP. Radiation colitis and proctitis. Clinics in Colon and Rectal Surgery. 2007;**20**:64-72

[23] McCrone LF, Neary PM, Larkin J, et al. The surgical management of radiation proctopathy. International Journal of Colorectal Disease. 2017;**32**:1099-1108

[24] Garg AK, Mai WY, McGary JE, et al. Radiation proctopathy in the treatment of prostate cancer. International Journal of Radiation Oncology, Biology, Physics. 2006;**66**:1294-1305

[25] Chruscielewska-Kiliszek MR, Rupinski M, Kraszewska E, et al. The protective role of antiplatelet treatment against ulcer formation due to argon plasma coagulation in patients treated for chronic radiation proctitis. Colorectal Disease. 2014;**16**:293-297

[26] Denham JW, O'Brien PC, Dunstan RH, et al. Is there more than one late radiation proctitis syndrome? Radiotherapy and Oncology. 1999;**51**:43-53

[27] Andreyev HJN, Wotherspoon A, Denham JW, et al. "Pelvic radiation disease": New understanding and new solutions for a new disease in the era of cancer survivorship. Scandinavian Journal of Gastroenterology. 2011;**46**:389-397

[28] Hayne D, Vaizey CJ, Boulos PB. Anorectal injury following pelvic radiotherapy. The British Journal of Surgery. 2001;**88**:1037-1048

[29] Nasierowska-Guttmejer A. Changes in the gastrointestinal mucosa after radio- and chemotherapy of the neoplasms. Oncology Review. 2012;**2**:39-44

[30] Takemoto S, Shibamoto Y, Ayakawa S, et al. Treatment and prognosis of patients with late rectal bleeding after intensity-modulated radiation therapy for prostate cancer. Radiation Oncology. 2012;**7**:87

[31] Leiper K, Morris AI. Treatment of radiation proctitis. Clinical Oncology. 2007;**19**:724-729

[32] Kim TG, Huh SJ, Park W. Endoscopic findings of rectal mucosal damage after pelvic radiotherapy for cervical carcinoma: Correlation of rectal mucosal damage with radiation dose and clinical symptoms. Journal of Radiation Oncology. 2013;**31**:81-87

[33] Shadad AK, Sullivan FJ, Martin JD, et al. Gastrointestinal radiation injury: Symptoms, risk factors and mechanisms. World Journal of Gastroenterology. 2013;**19**(2):185-198

[34] Andreyev HJN, Benton BE, Lalji A, et al. Algorithm-based management of patients with gastrointestinal symptoms in patients after pelvic radiation treatment (ORBIT): A randomised controlled trial. Lancet. 2013;**382**:2084-2092

[35] Andreyev J. Gastrointestinal symptoms after pelvic radiotherapy: A new understanding to improve management of symptomatic patients. The Lancet Oncology. 2007;**8**:1007-1017

[36] Andreyev HJN. Pelvic radiation disease. Colorectal Disease. 2015;**17**:2-6

[37] Goldner G, Tomicek B, Becker G, et al. Proctitis after external-beam radiotherapy for prostate cancer classified by Vienna rectoscopy score and correlated with EORTC/RTOG score for late rectal toxicity: Results of a prospective multicenter study of 166 patients. International Journal of Radiation Oncology, Biology, Physics. 2007;**67**:78-83

[38] Wachter S, Gerstner N, Goldner G, et al. Endoscopic scoring of late rectal mucosal damage after conformal radiotherapy for prostatic carcinoma. Radiotherapy and Oncology. 2000;**54**:11-19

[39] McElvanna K, Wilson A, Irwin T. Sucralfate paste enema: A new method of topical treatment for haemorrhagic radiation proctitis. Colorectal Disease. 2014;**16**:281-284

[40] Ma TH, Yuan ZH, Zhong QH, et al. Formalin irrigation for hemorrhagic chronic radiation proctitis. World Journal of Gastroenterology. 2015;**21**(12):3593-3598

[41] Wong MTC, Lim JF, Ho KS, et al. Radiation proctitis: A decade's experience. Singapore Medical Journal. 2010;**51**:315-319

[42] Eifel PJ, Levenback C, Wharton JT, et al. Time course and incidence of late complications in patients treated with radiation therapy for FIGO Stage IB carcinoma of the uterine cervix. International Journal of Radiation Oncology, Biology, Physics. 1995;**32**:1289-1300

[43] O'Brien PC, Hamilton C, Denham JW. Spontaneous improvement in late rectal mucosal changes after radiotherapy for prostate cancer. International Journal of Radiation Oncology, Biology, Physics. 2004;**58**:75-80

[44] Gilinsky NH, Burns DG, Barbezat GO, et al. The natural history of radiation-induced proctosigmoiditis: An analysis of 88 patients. The Quarterly Journal of Medicine, New Series LII. 1983;**205**(Winter):40-53

[45] Craanen ME, van Triest B, Verheijen RHM, et al. Thalidomide in refractory haemorrhagic radiation induced proctitis. Gut. 2006;**55**:1371-1372

[46] Hopkins JC, Wood JJ, Gilbert H, et al. Trans-anal rectoscopic ball diathermy (TARD) for radiotherapy-induced haemorrhagic telangiectasia: A safe and effective treatment. Colorectal Disease. 2013;**15**:566-568

[47] Hou JK, Abudayyeh A, Shaib Y. Treatment of chronic radiation proctitis with cryoablation. Gastrointestinal Endoscopy. 2011;**73**:383-389

[48] Hauer-Jensen M, Wang J, Denham JW. Bowel injury: Current and evolving management strategies. Seminars in Radiation Oncology. 2003;**13**:357-371

[49] Sudha AP, Kadambari D. Efficacy and safety of argon plasma coagulation in the management of extensive chronic radiation proctitis after pelvic radiotherapy for cervical carcinoma. International Journal of Colorectal Disease. 2017;**32**:1285-1288

[50] Hoggan BL, Cameron AL. Systematic review of hyperbaric oxygen therapy for the treatment of non-neurological soft tissue radiation-related injuries. Support Care Cancer. 2014;**22**:1715-1726

[51] Takeuchi H, Kimura T, Okamoto K, et al. A mechanism for abnormal angiogenesis in human radiation proctitis: analysis of expression profile for angiogenic factors. Journal of Gastroenterology. 2012;**47**:56-64

Section 5

Fecal Incontinence

Chapter 7

Faecal Incontinence

Filippo La Torre and Diego Coletta

Additional information is available at the end of the chapter

http://dx.doi.org/10.5772/intechopen.77393

Abstract

Fecal incontinence (FI) is an extremely common condition, whose true prevalence is difficult to assess. It was defined as the uncontrolled passage of fecal material recurring for >3 months. Fecal incontinence is related to many etiologic factors, but one of the most frequent causes is secondary to pelvic and/or anal and rectal surgery, childbirth-related damage, or other pelvic trauma. Fecal incontinence after surgery may be elicited by many pelvic, rectal, and anal surgical/obstetric procedures, which contribute through different mechanisms to incontinence. After accurate evaluation, the first line approach with medical and behavioral treatments often fails in treating FI. Rehabilitative therapy and less invasive procedures are preferred before performing standard surgical intervention, while invasive procedures are to be discouraged.

Keywords: fecal incontinence, anorectal manometry, endoanal ultrasound, bulking agents, sphincteroplasty

1. Introduction

Fecal incontinence (FI) is an extremely common condition, whose true prevalence is difficult to assess. It was defined as the uncontrolled passage of fecal material recurring for >3 months [1]. The employment of absorbent pads, alimentary restriction, and other restraint principals, up until the last few years, was the only treatment within nonspecialized centers. One of the side effects of dysfunctional sphincter is the inability to hold gas and feces. Incontinence is the result of irregularity of any of the systems, anatomic and neurophysiological structures, together with other systemic diseases, which may have altered intestinal motility and stool consistency as well as diseases that affect superior cerebral capability. Incontinence reduces significantly the patient's quality of life and leads patients to renounce all forms of social daily life. With the passing of the years, changes in pelvic floor structures, connective tissue, smooth and striated muscle component lead to an increase in prevalence of the incontinence. The psycho-emotional effects, namely, stress, anguish, tears, anxiety, fatigue, fear of public humiliation, and the sensation to be dirty and smelling are devastating. Limited sexual activity is inevitable as also fear of the anticipated incontinence, fury, abasement, depression, insulation, and frustration. In addition, activity is seriously impaired; for many patients, trivially walking can be a time to deal with unpleasant inconveniences and that results in avoiding every daily activities. After accurate evaluation, the first line approach with medical and behavioral treatments often fails in treating FI. Rehabilitative therapy and less invasive procedures are preferred before performing standard surgical intervention, while invasive procedures are to be discouraged.

2. Fecal incontinence following surgery or trauma

Fecal incontinence is related to many etiologic factors, but one of the most frequent causes is secondary to pelvic and/or anal and rectal surgery, childbirth-related damage or other pelvic trauma. Fecal incontinence after surgery may be elicited by many pelvic, rectal, and anal surgical/obstetric procedures, which contribute through different mechanisms to incontinence. Until quite recently, the surgical management of fecal incontinence has, for almost 25 years, focused on the repair of injuries sustained to the anal sphincter complex. The advent of anal ultrasound in the late 1980s allows better case selection through improved recognition and characterization of anterior obstetric and anal defects amenable to repair, previously relied only to clinical examination [2].

3. Clinical assessment

Medical, surgical and obstetric history is the first attempt to evaluate a patient suffering from fecal incontinence. Information regarding stool form according to the Bristol scale [1, 3], number of bowel movements/week, pathological pre-existing conditions and procedures of former rectal and/or anal surgery were collected from previous outpatient charts. The surgical operations were categorized according to type of surgical procedure, operation date, underlying disease, time elapsed between surgical procedure and outpatient observation. Obstetric trauma has the highest incidence, both following a surgical procedure (episiotomy) and a sequel of traumatic delivery (prolonged labor, a disproportion between the size of the baby and the pelvis, breech delivery, forceps use). The Sultan classification [4] has been adopted by the International Consultation on Incontinence [5] and the Royal of obstetricians and gynecologists. Different scores are used to classify fecal incontinence: Fecal Incontinence Severity Index (FISI) score [6], Fecal incontinence quality of life (FIQL) [7], Rapid assessment fecal incontinence score (RAFIS) [8], Gastrointestinal Quality of Life Index (GIQLI) [9], and Wexner and Jorge scale [10]. Rectal examination remains the first attempt to evaluate the condition of anal sphincter in patients with FI, showing good sensitivity and poor specificity in discerning small from severe global anal sphincter defects. Moreover, digital rectal examination had fair sensitivity and poor specificity in grading external anal sphincter defects, and its best accuracy was on complete external anal sphincter lesions. Anal resting and squeeze tone were correlated to anal pressures [11].

4. Diagnosis

4.1. Functional tests

4.1.1. Anorectal manometry

A useful functional test for accurate definition of anal canal pressures, recto-anal inhibitory reflex, rectal sensations and rectal compliance is anorectal-manometry (ARM). Fecal incontinence is evaluated using all these parameters. Different methods to acquire data regarding ARM in FI management are employed: classic water perfusion manometry, solid-state manometry [12], and high-resolution manometry [13, 14]. Solid-state probe with strain gauge transducers or water-perfused probes is actually in use. A central lumen ends in a 4-cm long, compliant balloon attached to the extremity of the catheter, at 4 cm from the distal recording point [12, 15, 16]. The water perfused manometry systems use pneumohydraulic pumps ensuring a rate of 0.2–0.4 ml/min with a pressure head of 10 psi. The sonde is introduced leaving pressure sensors and balloon in the rectum, and a rest time of 5 min is necessary to allow the anal basal tone to become again to its starting value. The resting anal pressure may be measured with a station pull-through technique withdrawing the probe step-by-step 0.5 cm at the time to record the pressure profile of the anal canal. If the patient is not totally at relax, there could be a stronger concurrence of the striated muscles and higher pressures certainly would be registered. Therefore, in order to obtain steady values, it would be preferable to place the sensors inside the anal canal and register the pressure at rest for longer period (5–15 min).

The basal tone is given by tonic activities of the internal anal sphincter (IAS) and of the external anal sphincter (EAS). Works on the effect of the IAS myotomy, general anesthesia [17], and of the block of pudendal nerve [18] on the anal pressures show that 75–85% of the rest pressure derives from the IAS and the remaining part from the EAS. To assess the strength and length of the voluntary contraction, the gauge sonde is positioned in the anal canal with registration bores in the high-pressure area, and the patient is asked to squeeze (≥2 attempts). The average of the highest pressures recorded at any site in the anal canal is used to calculate the maximum squeeze pressure [12, 16]. The duration of squeezing can be intended as the period in which the squeeze pressure is maintained above 50% of the maximum value or as the interval between the beginning of the pressure increasing in the anal canal and the pressure curve returns to the starting values. The squeeze maneuver assesses the function and the voluntary control of the EAS. Recent works, using manometry and 3D ultrasound of the anal canal [19], reported the association between increased pressure along the entire anal canal and the contraction of puborectalis muscle and EAS. These data suggest that the puborectalis muscle takes parts to the squeezing time in the proximal portion of the anal canal, while the EAS in the distal portion and the maximal values are registered where the puborectalis overlaps EAS. Involuntary contraction of the EAS occurs during blunt change in abdominal pressure: this is a multisynaptic sacral reflex that prevents anal incontinence in such conditions and that is voluntarily inhibited during defecation. To check the integrity of this reflex, the patient is invited to make a cough: this reflex response results in the anal sphincter pressure to rise above that of the rectum. The cough reflex is evaluated as the highest positive difference between the increases of the anal pressure in comparison with the increase of the rectal pressure in two attempts [12]. Picking at the perianal skin is possible to attend at a contraction of EAS: this is the anocutaneous reflex. Anal pressures vary by age and sex even though there exists a sizable overlapping in values [15, 16, 20, 21]. Measured pressures tend to be higher when you run a quick pull-through [10]. Barostat test would be the ideal method for assessing the sensorial and viscoelastic characteristics of the rectum, even though it is still use in routinely valuation because of its cost. During ARM, a balloon is inflated in the rectum with increasing volumes of air to keep some information over the viscoelastic properties and sensory functions. This procedure is less accurate than the detailed barostat test, but it is considered sufficient to keep information about clinical rectal properties. The rectal balloon is intermittently air inflated. Each inflation is performed every 30–60 s and implies a 10 ml volume gain up to 200 ml of air or the beginning of pain/discomfort. The rectal balloon is completely deflated after each step [12, 16]. Rectum responds to filling with visceral relaxation for comfortably storing feces until the voluntary defecation: this accommodation is described by the rectal compliance, which is a volume/pressure curve. The pressure in the balloon during the distension seems to be connected to the internal rectal pressure, and its recording is used to assess the rectal compliance. The balloon inflation causes a fast increasing of the balloon pressure, followed by a decline to a steady-state value as the rectum fits to the increased volume. The rectal steady state is calculated as the difference between the recorded pressure and the pressure obtained during the inflation of the balloon. High compliance rates means that the rectum has excessive relaxation and then results in poor increased pressure in its lumen, conversely low compliance rates describe a poor adaptation of the rectum to volume gains and then results in high intra-rectal pressures. The distension of the rectum by increasing volumes is aimed also to evaluate rectal sensibility. The patient is invited to refer the feelings in the rectum. Usually, three steps of sensations are identified: (1) feeling of fullness or distention, (2) steady bid to evacuate, and (3) maximum tolerable volume that can be associated with painful sensation [12, 16]. Large size and/or high compliant rectum requires large volume to evoke the call to evacuate; in noncompliant rectum, small volume can induce urgency [22]. However, balloon inflections used to assess the rectal compliance and sensibility seem to have some limits: in addition to the fact, the rectum is an open cavity, the results depend on both technique and operator. Recorded data may vary according to the size and the nature of the balloon and the method of air inflation and its velocity. The rectal sensibility can also be modified by the discomfort caused by the maneuver and/or by the use of clyster before the test. Distention of the rectum causes a transitory decrement of the basal anal pressure due to the relaxation of the IAS: this characteristic is known as the rectoanal inhibitory reflex (RAIR). It is a reflex mediated via the myenteric plexus. It can be also identified as a "sampling mechanism" to discriminate the rectal content: flatus and consistence of feces. The characteristics of the RAIR depend on some technical aspects: the rectum should be empty, megarectum needs high volume to reach the correct level of distension in order to evocate the reflex, the pressure drop can be obscured by the EAS contraction, or it cannot be evident at all when the resting pressure is very low. The nondetectability of RAIR is diagnostic for Hirschsprung's disease with a sensitivity of 91% and specificity of 94%. In constipated patients, it is convenient to evaluate the defecatory maneuver. The patient is invited to defecate to evaluate sphincter responses during the maneuver, while the rectal balloon can be inflated with air or water. Normal pattern should result in increasing the internal rectal pressure, which is synergic with the decrease in the internal anal pressure. Some patients may have anal pressure increment during straining for the paradoxical contraction of the EAS or lack of anal relaxation: in both cases, there is an obstacle to evacuate [12]. In a third pattern of dyssynergic defecation, the internal rectal pressure is lower than anal pressure [12]. The maneuver can be altered by outpatient condition (position of the patient, lack of privacy); actually, it is poorly reproducible and altered patterns are recorded also in asymptomatic subjects. Anorectal manometry is suggested in the workup for fecal incontinence because it provides objective assessment of the anal sphincter function. The manometric parameters usually considered are resting pressure, squeeze pressure, rectal compliance, and rectal sensibility.

4.1.2. *Electromyography*

Another functional evaluation is the anal neurophysiological testing. External anal sphincter electromyography, motor-evoked potentials, somatosensory evoked potentials, and sacral anal reflex latency measurement are currently available to evaluate neurogenic anorectal disorders. Pudendal nerve supplies voluntary control of external anal sphincter, diagnosis of its damage may be reached with neurophysiological tests and a prolongation of electrical impulse across it may have several impacts on evacuative control [23]. Finally, anal electromyography may be helpful in patients with obstructed defecation. It senses electrical activity during rest, squeeze, and strain and can be useful to identify patients with paradoxical contraction of the puborectalis, sign of pelvic floor dyssynergia.

5. Imaging

5.1. Endoanal ultrasound

Endoanal ultrasound allows to visualize the complete ring of the internal anal sphincter (IAS), the complete ring of the superficial external anal sphincter (EAS) (concentric band of mixed echogenicity) and the thickness of both anal sphincters in the middle level of the anal canal [24, 25]. A discontinuity of the muscle, with an area of mixed echogenicity due to replacement of muscle cells by fibrous tissue, was read as a defect of IAS or EAS. The sphincter defect was measured in degrees. Diffuse thinning and/or replacement of muscle fibers by fat defined external anal sphincter atrophy. Internal anal sphincter atrophy was identified as diffuse thinning of the sphincter. Correct acquaintance of the normal ultrasonographic anatomy of the anal canal is necessary to identify abnormalities. In particular, EAUS is currently the gold standard exam for internal and external anal sphincter defects identification in fecal incontinence. Most recent studies showed 80–100% sensitivity in identifying sphincter's damages. Endosonographic scanning is performed with a 7 or 10 MHz rotating endoprobe, providing a 360° axial view of the anal canal; three-dimensional endosonography allows multiplanar imaging of the anal sphincters. Color or power Doppler imaging technology can also be used with endosonography [26]. The examination is performed with the patient placed in the left lateral position, in the knee-chest position. A digital anorectal examination must be performed before the insertion of the probe to visualize the lesion's size and location and the status of the anal sphincters [27, 28]. At the moment of the insertion of the probe into the anal canal, it is usually put in line with standard orientation, in which the anterior anatomical structures are at the uppermost or 12 o'clock side of the image, the patient's left side is at 3 o'clock, the patient's posterior side is at 6 o'clock, and the patient's right side is at 9 o'clock. To cover the entire length of the anorectal canal, the probe should be introduced up to 8–9 cm, approximately at the level of peritoneal reflection. Then, the probe is slowly retracted, and images are obtained at different levels through the anal canal [29].

The anatomy of the anal sphincter complex is based on four layers: (1) sub-epithelial tissues (medium reflectivity), (2) IAS – hypoechoic (low reflectivity), (3) the longitudinal-muscle layer (variable reflectivity), (4) EAS – hyperechoic (variable reflectivity).

The anal canal is conventionally divided into three different parts: (1) upper anal canal which is a hyperechoic horseshoe sling of the puborectalis muscle posteriorly and loss of the EAS in the midline anteriorly; (2) middle anal canal level which is the completion of the EAS ring anteriorly in combination with the maximum IAS thickness (IAS is seen as a hypoechoic ring-like structure); (3) the lower anal canal level is defined as that immediately caudal to the termination of the IAS and comprises the subcutaneous EAS. Moreover, the IAS gets slightly thicker, and the EAS gets thinner with increasing age. It is important to consider some snares in the reading of EAS images. The female anterior EAS anatomically situated below the level of the puborectalis sling may be wrongly interpreted as an anterior EAS damage. The anococcygeal ligament, with its triangular hypoechoic structure on the axial images posteriorly, should not be confused with a sphincter defect. On endoanal sonography, atrophic or degenerative sphincters are seen as thin and poorly defined and often with heterogeneous increased echogenicity. Increased echogenicity on endoanal sonography has been shown histologically to be correlated with replacement of smooth muscle by fibrous tissue. It will be important to recognize abnormal thinning and physiologic age-related EAS differences. This should be a problem in the EAS because the EAS muscle is also thinner at older ages, and it may be difficult to distinguish sufficiently between atrophy and age-related changes [30]. The IAS is very clearly seen on endoanal sonography, and it is easier to appreciate atrophy and small tears of this sphincter. Moreover, 3D endoanal sonography facilitates sagittal and coronal reconstruction of the anal canal, resulting in better delineation of the normal anatomy and defects of the anal sphincter. On endoanal sonography, scar tissue seems to be a mixed echogenic area. A discontinuity of the anal sphincters results as a localized defect. The localized defect of the IAS appears as hyperechoic break, and EAS tears appear as relatively hypoechoic areas. An injury of the EAS due to vaginal delivery is typically anterior, usually in the right anterolateral side. In contrast, an isolated IAS injury almost never follows childbirth and indicates a primary traumatic cause from within the anal canal, most commonly surgical interventions. During the exam should be carefully registered the number, the circumferential and the longitudinal extent of all defects. Anal sphincter injury related to vaginal delivery in female is the most common cause of fecal incontinence due to direct or indirect anal sphincter muscles damage or sphincter innervation. They are identified in 0.6–9.0% of vaginal deliveries where mediolateral episiotomy is performed, but the detection in EAUS is much higher. Typically, anal sphincter defects childbirth related are ultrasonically seen as an interruption of the normal U-shaped, upper—or round—middle, and low aspect of the EAS characterized by a "loss" of the right anterolateral arm of the EAS (from 9 o'clock to 11 o'clock) because the episiotomy is usually realized, by a right-hander gynecologist, in this anterolateral area. If the EAUS after vaginal delivery will detect an important anal sphincter defect—even little symptomatic—it should be immediately repaired to decrease the risk of severe FI. Anorectal surgery represents the second most frequent cause of sphincter lesion. In all cases of anorectal surgery, especially in cases of a procedure with more risk of postsurgical sphincter lesions—fistula in ano—and even for simple anorectal surgery, as in the case of a patient who is multiparous or with previous perianal surgery or trauma, EAUS is mandatory to be performed to evaluate the status of the sphincter complex to avoid surgical procedures that could make unmask a preexisting sphincter incontinence in the postoperative period. When a hemorrhoidectomy or a prolapsectomy is performed, respectively, the removal of hemorrhoidal cushions or the postoperative fecal urgency that can occur after prolapsectomy can improve a light or subclinical fecal incontinence [31]. Moreover, an anal sphincterotomy performed for anal fissure could became the final act responsible for moving a previous asymptomatic sphincter lesion in a clinical fecal incontinence. In particular, EAUS in patients surgically treated for anal fissure might show insufficient sphincterotomy and sphincterial thickening because of the persistence of fissure and anal pain or, on the contrary, demonstrate an excessive sphincterotomy with temporary or permanent incontinence. In case of a surgery for fistula in ano, an endoanal US should be performed in the preoperative for mapping the abscess and identify the fistula, but also to exclude the presence of a previous internal, external, or both sphincter lesions. This relief could change the quality and outcome of surgery [32]. The preoperative EAUS is, however, recommended for every fistula because the fistula that was preoperatively judged easy might demonstrate as complex at surgery or at the postoperative follow-up with potential even dramatic sphincter consequences [33, 34]. In recurrent or complex fistula in ano, 3D EAUS (sometimes with hydrogen peroxide) proved to be more accurate than 2D for detecting difficult (hidden) primary or secondary tracks and internal openings [35]. It should be underlined, however, that an endoanal US realized in an operated patient could offer important difficulties of interpretation of the US images for the presence of fibrosclerotic tissue and/or artifacts.

5.2. Magnetic resonance imaging in fecal incontinence

An imaging assessment is mandatory in evaluating anal incontinence as sphincter tears are overlooked at clinical examination. Loss of ring continuity and loss of homogeneous intensity signal of the sphincters are pathologic detections due to damage of muscle fibers. Breakage of the normal shape with hypointense alteration of the muscle fibers is pathognomonic of the presence of scar tissue. It is visible as hypointense tissue because of its content in fibrous tissue, more hypointense than the normal external sphincter, distorting the normal multilayered architecture of the sphincter muscle. Fat replacement is also a finding consistent with atrophy even if the sphincter thickness is preserved [36]. Many studies have demonstrated that despite its lower local spatial resolution, external phase-array MR imaging is comparable to endoanal magnetic resonance imaging (MRI) for the depiction of anal sphincter defects and EAS atrophy. Endoanal exam have limits as the discomfort in the introduction of the coil, the reduced quality of images due to artifacts from movement and interface between the probe and the rectum, and probable stretching of the sphincter muscles caused by the probe itself with consequent underestimation of their thickness [37, 38]. External phased-array MRI imaging has demonstrated atrophy of EAS in most women complaining fecal incontinence and an IAS defect in women with previous obstetric trauma. Besides external phased-array MRI can identify other defects of pelvic floor structures. Puborectalis muscle atrophy, shown as an abnormal thinning, has also been found in a considerable number of fecal incontinent patients. Pubo-rectalis and levator-ani muscle defects are relatively common in women with severe fecal incontinence, however usually associated to sphincter injury than solitary defects. MRI has demonstrated that levator-ani muscle injury is present in lot of women with EAS injuries who delivered vaginally, and those women patients were frequently suffering from fecal incontinence. Anorectal angle (ARA) change during squeeze was lower in subjects with fecal incontinence who had a history of a third- or fourth degree perineal tear, indicating a lower function of the pubo-rectalis muscle [39]. It is important to assess the sphincter integrity with MRI because patients who have only a focal defect may benefit from surgical repair [40], or in the case of incontinence and rectal prolapse, patients may achieve restoration of continence after rectopexy [41]. In the selection of patients for anal sphincter repair, both endoanal MR and endoanal sonography are sensitive tools for pre-operatory assessment, but endoanal MRI is capable of depicting EAS atrophy, with a sensitivity of 81% and a positive predictive value of 89% compared to surgical findings, which is associated with a poor outcome of anterior anal sphincter repair [42, 43]. Patients with external sphincter atrophy at a preoperatory assessment have worse outcome after repair, while those with normal external thickness show a better postsurgical outcome [44]. MRI defecography (dynamic imaging of the pelvic floor) has also been evaluated in selecting surgical options in anal incontinence and MRI defecography reveals various pelvic floor abnormalities including rectal descent, cystocele, enterocele, rectocele, and rectal invagination. Moreover, 50% of patients revealed ARA changes <10% between rest and squeezing and rest and defecation, indicating a dysfunction of puborectalis sling mechanism. Experience of radiologist is important in evaluating the sphincters complex, being the interobserver agreement stronger if both internal and external sphincters are intact or damaged [45]. MRI provides an accurate depiction of anal sphincter complex and pelvic floor anatomy with evaluation of muscle integrity and being a valuable tool to assess functional abnormalities of the pelvic floor as well. Either endoanal or external MRI can be used to evaluate muscle integrity with comparable results. External phased-array MRI provides information on pelvic floor muscle, while dynamic imaging is an additional tool to assess if pelvic floor prolapsed (bladder, uterine, or rectal) is associated. These information are of main diagnostic importance in evaluating fecal incontinence and aid treatment decision-making.

6. Treatment

The first step of therapy is conservative approaches, especially in patients with mild symptomatology, as dietary changing, medical therapy, muscles exercises (*exercises of Kegel*), biofeedback, and nonsurgical electrical nerve stimulation. Dietary changing avoiding caffeine, fruits rich on fibers, spicy foods, alcohol, and milky products (in patients with lactose intolerance) may help, but evidence on these restrictions is lacking. Smoking and sedentary lifestyle can be associated with FI [46].

6.1. Kinesitherapy

Kinesitherapy is a rehabilitative method that alleviates symptoms and obtains the greatest possible recovery of lost or altered function, by utilizing therapeutic exercise and movement of the body or part of it to treat disease [47]. Pelviperineal kinesitherapy or pelvic floor muscle training (PFMT) occupies a very important position in rehabilitation in the fields of urogynecology and proctology. PFMT typically consists of verbally guided instruction in pelvic floor and sphincter contractions (*Kegel contractions*). Anal sphincter exercises are performed to strengthen the puborectalis muscle, which is continuous with the external anal sphincter [48]. The technique is to consider pelvic floor like an elevator that can stop at different floors as it can go up and down. Other reported methods include working on coordination of anal sphincter activity and working to isolate a contraction of the anal sphincter. Some therapists use to place an hand externally or to guide the patient with finger placed vaginally or rectally for the correct exercise techniques, but most would argue that this constitutes a form of low-tech biofeedback training. Biofeedback therapy (BFB) includes many different types of training exercises for the pelvic floor. Biofeedback is defined as the process of gaining greater awareness of many physiological functions, primarily using instruments that provide information on the activity of those same systems, with a goal of being able to manipulate them at will. For pelvic floor rehabilitation purposes, the most common type of biofeedback is EMG that based on biofeedback therapy, which was introduced in 1979 [49]. Biofeedback is performed using visual, auditory, or verbal feedback techniques with an anorectal manometer or electromyographic sonde inserted into the rectum to display pressure modifications [50]. Data are registered either through surface electrodes or via the use of intravaginal or intrarectal sensors. Electrical stimulation is another modality that has been used for the rehabilitative therapy of FI. The target of electrical stimulation is to improve the strength and/or endurance of striated muscles contraction with the objective being typically identified with the external anal sphincter. Another goal can be to allow patients with decreased kinesthetic awareness to become more cognizant of where their pelvic floor muscles are in space and what it feels like when the muscles and sphincter are contracting. Electrical stimulation can be delivered to the pelvic floor and anal sphincter in many different forms, including via surface electrodes or intrarectal probes and with many different stimulation parameters and treatment protocols. All forms of electrical stimulation are often used with PFMT or biofeedback training, although stimulation can be used alone as rehabilitative treatment. Transcutaneous and percutaneous tibial nerve stimulations have been tried in patients with FI. In a randomized, double-blind, sham- controlled trial, 144 patients were randomly assigned to receive either active or sham stimulations for 3 months. No statistically significant difference was shown between real and sham transcutaneous electrical nerve stimulation (TENS) in terms of an improvement in the number of FI/urgency episodes per week [51].

6.2. Sacral nerve stimulation

Anorectal and pelvic floor innervation derive from the autonomic and the somatic nervous systems. Motor innervation of the levator-ani muscle and pubo-rectalis sling starts in the sacral nerve roots (S2–S5) [52–54]. The EAS is innervated by a branch of the pudendal nerve, the inferior rectal nerve [52]. Autonomic innervation is sympathetic and parasympathetic. Parasympathetic innervation is through the pelvic plexus, derived from the sacral nerves (S2–S4) [52]. Anal and distal rectal sensory innervation is mainly through the pudendal nerve [55]. Electrical stimulation of this dual innervation seems to excite both systems and causes both direct and reflex-mediated responses in the fecal continence mechanism [56, 57]. The real mechanism of action of SNS in the treatment of bowel and urinary dysfunctions is not cleared yet. The great part of the studies was conducted in patients affected by urinary dysfunctions. For infants, who have not yet achieved voluntary control, a critical level of bladder distention is required to stimulate the voiding reflex. This sensory input, on reaching the pontine micturition center, simultaneously allows for a coordinated detrusor contraction and concomitant urethral relaxation. Gaining voluntary control, the voiding reflex becomes a complex process mediated at a higher level in the cerebral cortex. Voluntary voiding is a result of inhibition of the sympathetic system and activation of the sacral parasympathetic system [58, 59]. In patients with fecal incontinence, limited information is available to explain the mechanism of action. A small study demonstrated that SNS was associated with higher tolerance of rectal distention, but the neurologic mechanism behind this is unclear [60]. Probably, the pudendal afferent somatic fibers work by inhibiting colonic propulsive activity and activating the internal anal sphincter [61]. The action on colonic motility may explain why patients with significant anal sphincter defects may benefit from SNS.

6.3. Injectable/implantable bulking agents

Injectable agents have been used for the first time as a treatment for urinary incontinence (UI), with the advantages of an ambulatory procedure and low morbidity rate but with variable success. Thereafter, different injectable agents have been employed for FI. The use of bulking agents in patients with FI is still controversial, mostly because of conflicting results and lack of agreement regarding adequate indications. Moreover, different techniques of injection have been performed, and several agents have been used via injection: Fat, PTQ®, Durasphere®, Coaptite®, NASHA TM -Dx, Permacol®, and BulkamidTM. Different techniques of delivery have been described, providing a submucosal injection inside the anal canal, intersphincteric or within the sphincter defect scar tissue; transanal/transmucosal, transsphincteric or intersphincteric were the route of injection at different areas of the anal canal, in two/three/four or more points [62–66].

Recently, a novel approach has been introduced to treat patients with FI, by the placement of implantable agents, in the form of thin cylinders, within the sphincteric complex. The THD Gatekeeper TM was the first device used, but very recently, the THD SphinKeeperTM has been available for procedure. Gatekeeper TM implants are made of a material (HYEXPAN TM) that is both solid at the time of delivery and slowly absorbs water to expand itself once implanted. Within 48 h, the implant should have reached its definitive size and shape. At this step, the consistency of the material has moved from hard to soft with shape memory, giving the implant a pliable texture that makes it compliant to external pressures without losing its original shape. For these reasons, it was decided to place the implants in the intersphincteric space, in the belief that this would achieve a more effective distribution of a presumed "bulking effects" than would be achieved with submucosal positioning, thus exploiting the physical characteristic of the implant most effectively. However, the "bulking effects" should be not the only and/or main effect contributing to the therapeutic efficacy. The intersphincteric location should also minimize the potential risk of erosion, ulceration, fistulation of the anal canal, and possible displacement of the prosthesis [67–70].

6.4. Artificial bowel sphincter

The artificial bowel sphincter (ABS together with dynamic graciloplasty and sacral nerve stimulation (SNS)) is still considered an optional treatment for refractory conservative treatment and severe fecal incontinence. Christiansen and Lorentzen first reported in 1987 a perianal implantation of an adapted artificial urinary sphincter (AMS 800, America Medical System) for a patient with fecal incontinence [71]. In 1996, Lehur and colleagues described the results obtained with an artificial bowel sphincter designed just for FI (Acticon Neosphincter – American Medical System) [72]. To date, despite the good results reported in the literature, in terms of improved continence and quality of life, the rate of surgical explantation and surgical procedures for infections of ABS still remains too high [73]. These were the reasons that reduced a wide acceptance of ABS in coloproctology practice. In accordance with Wexner et al., the cumulative risk of device explant increases with time but less dramatically in the longer follow-up [74]. Moreover, Wong et al. have shown, in long-term follow-up, as after explantation for infection the reimplantation can be performed without difficulty [75].

ABS implantation represents the last resort after failure of conservative and less-invasive surgical procedures in fecal incontinence [76]. It is indicated especially in patients with almost complete sphincter damage or post-surgical sphincter excision or for patients with congenital malformation or with significant neurological dysfunction [77]. In order to achieve long-term satisfying results and to use the device completely and competently, potential candidates must not have recent or active perineal infection and should not have manual limitations [78, 79]. Artificial sphincter was used before for treating urinary incontinence and later modified for fecal incontinence. The ABS, Acticon Neosphincter (American Medical Systems, Minnetonka, MN, USA) aims to control incontinence by mimicking the natural action of the sphincter muscle. The device composed of three parts: an inflatable cuff that works as the new sphincter and seals the anal canal, a control pump, and a pressure-regulating balloon that also functions as a fluid reservoir connected by two special tubes system [80]. The patient is placed in the lithotomy position under general anesthesia. The cuff is positioned creating a tunnel around the rectum; the balloon is implanted ahead to the bladder in the Retzius space and the pump is inserted into the major labia in women or inside the scrotum in men [79, 81, 82].

6.5. Reconstructive surgery

Reconstructive surgery is indicated more specifically in cases of fecal incontinence incurred by anal sphincter lesions, abnormalities, or deformities, as well as sphincter deficiency with no evident lesions and abnormalities of the pelvic floor.

The following are several reconstructive techniques:

- Sphincteroplasty.
- Suture of the levator ani.
- Reconstruction of the sphincter complex using muscle repair.

Surgical techniques which resulting in a direct repair are only indicated for lesions located in the external anal sphincter. The main cause of sphincter lesions is obstetric trauma. Despite the lack of any particular continence consequences caused by childbirth, 1–4% of deliveries result in lesions of the sphincter complex or of the pelvic floor (lesions of the third and fourth degrees) [83–86]. Fetus weight, surgical incision on the midline of the perineum (episiotomy), the use of forceps, and breech presentation are considered the main risk factors of sphincter damage [87–89]. Obstetric damages can be detected immediately in the postpartum and are caused by third degree laceration, but approximately in 40% of cases [88], continence dysfunctions are detected as early as 6 months post-delivery [85]. The most frequently performed surgical procedure for the treatment of obstetric lesions is direct anterior sphincter suture repair [89]. Optimal timing for the repair is within 3–4 months following the trauma. Anal sphincter repair can be performed using the "end-to-end" technique, thereby facing the two laps after resecting scar tissue as well as through the "overlapping" technique, which is performed by overlaying the residual functional extremities. The first technique is used to repair recent injuries in which the scar that has outdistanced the extremities of the muscles is not yet formed, thus allowing for the facing of the extremities without excessive tension. In old injuries, the sphincter defect is often consolidated, and a direct suture of the extremities is to be avoided at all cost, as it would be invariably destined to failure. The overlapping technique is generally quite safe for sphincter suture repair; suture repairs of the pelvic muscles, performed alone or with a sphincteroplasty, are carried out in order to treat muscle deficit or defects. The goal of this type of technique is the restoration of tension to the functionally deficient sphincter muscles through the use of plication. In the history of surgery, the first recommended and validated procedure was the postanal repair, presented by Parks in 1971 and subsequently modified [90]. This procedure was at first suggested to patients with neurogenic or idiopathic fecal incontinence, with no sphincter defect. The anterior levatorplasty procedure is often performed to treat pelvic trauma frequently resulting from obstetric injury. These types of surgical procedures are performed when an attempt to restore the sphincter using the aforementioned technique has not led to any effective results. The logic behind this strategy is to recreate the anal sphincter by replacing degenerative tissue with ectopic muscle located at the perineal level or by using a prosthetic device [91]. Muscle transposition and prosthetic replacement are two different techniques, yet both utilize the same functionality: to create an area with high pressure around the terminal part of the gastrointestinal tract by tightening around the distal rectum. Another option is the muscle of the lower limb, which extends from the ischium to the knee joint, also called "rectus femoris muscle" alternatively; the gluteus maximus muscle may be used. Dynamic graciloplasty is often indicated as the type of procedure with the most favorable outcomes, above all thanks to its anatomical characteristics that predispose its transposition [92].

6.6. Intestinal ostomy

When all surgical treatments fail, bowel ostomy may be considered an effective, safe, and appropriate surgical solution for patients with severe incontinence [93]. Indications for colostomy/ileostomy include spinal cord injury, complete pelvic floor denervation, severe perineal trauma, and actinic FI that can lead to severe neurogenic incontinence. It is performed on patients immobilized with skin problems or other complications too [94] or on those who are physically or mentally incapable without any bowel control resulting in a poor quality of life [95]. The creation of a colostomy or ileostomy provides definitive control of fecal incontinence. It is usually performed if other treatment options had no satisfying results. Patients are usually understandably very unwilling to the idea of a permanent ostomy, fearing it will be difficult to manage due to the great impact on self-image and social interactions.

Conflict of interest

The authors had no conflict of interest.

Author details

Filippo La Torre and Diego Coletta*

*Address all correspondence to: diegocoletta1@gmail.com

Unit of Emergency Surgery and Trauma, Policlinico Umberto I University Hospital, Sapienza University of Rome, Rome

References

[1] Pucciani F. Fecal soiling: Pathophysiology of postdefaecatory incontinence. Colorectal Disease. 2013;**15**:987-992

[2] Stergios DK. Childbirt Trauma. London: Springer Verlag Ltd; 2017. 329 p. DOI: 10.1007/978-1-4471-6711-2

[3] O'Donnell LJ, Virjee J, Heaton KW. Pseudo-diarrhoea in the irritable bowel syndrome: Patients' records of stool form reflect transit time while stool frequency does not. Gut. 1988;**29**:A1455

[4] Sultan AH. Obstetric perineal injury and anal incontinence. Clinical Risk. 1999;**5**(6):193-196

[5] Koelbl H, Igawa T, Salvatore S, Laterza RM, Lowry A, Sievert KD, et al. Pathophysiology of urinary incontinence, faecal incontinence and pelvic organ prolapse. In: Abrams P, Cardozo L, Khoury S, Wein A, editors. Incontinence. 5th ed. Paris: ICUDEAU; 2013. pp. 261-359

[6] Rockwood TH, Church JM, Fleshman JW, et al. Patient and surgeon ranking of the severity of symptoms associated with fecal incontinence: The fecal incontinence severity index. Diseases of the Colon and Rectum. 1999;**42**:1525-1532

[7] Rockwood TH, Church JM, Fleshman JW, Kane RL, Mavrantonis C, Thorson AG, Wexner SD, Bliss D, Lowry AC. Fecal incontinence quality of life scale: Quality of life instrument for patients with fecal incontinence. Diseases of the Colon and Rectum. 2000;**43**:9-16

[8] de la Portilla F, Calero-Lillo A, Jiménez-Rodríguez RM, Reyes ML, Segovia-González M, Maestre MV, García-Cabrera AM. Validation of a new scoring system: Rapid assessment faecal incontinence score. World Journal of Gastrointestinal Surgery. 2015 Sep 27;**7**(9):203-207

[9] Eypasch E, Williams JI, Wood-Dauphinee S, Ure BM, Schmulling C, Neugebauer E, Troidl H. Gastrointestinal quality of life index (development, validation and application of a new instrument). The British Journal of Surgery. 1995;**82**:216-222

[10] Jorge JM, Wexner SD. Etiology and management of fecal incontinence. Diseases of the Colon and Rectum. 1993;**36**:77-97

[11] Coura MM, Silva SM, Almeida RM, Forrest MC, Sousa JB. Is digital rectal exam reliable in grading anal sphincter defects. Archives of Gastroenterology. 2016 Oct-Dec;**53**(4):240-245

[12] Rao SS, Azpiroz F, Diamant N, et al. Minimum standards of anorectal manometry. Neurogastroenterology and Motility. 2002;**14**(5):553-559

[13] Rao SS. Advances in diagnostic assessment of fecal incontinence and dyssynergic defecation. Clinical Gastroenterology and Hepatology. 2010;**8**(11):910-919

[14] Jones MP, Post J, Crowell MD. High-resolution manometry in the evaluation of anorectal disorders: A simultaneous comparison with water-perfused manometry. The American Journal of Gastroenterology. 2007;**102**(4):850-855

[15] Rao SS, Hatfi eld R, Soffer E, et al. Manometric tests of anorectal function in healthy adults. The American Journal of Gastroenterology. 1999;**94**(3):773-783

[16] Gruppo Lombardo per lo Studio della Motilità Intestinale. Anorectal manometry with water- perfused catheter in healthy adults with no functional bowel disorders. Colorectal Disease. 2010;**12**:220-225

[17] Bennett RC, Duthie HL. The functional importance of the internal anal sphincter. The British Journal of Surgery. 1964;**51**(5):355-357

[18] Frenckner B, Euler CV. Influence of pudendal block on the function of the anal sphincters. Gut. 1975;**16**(6):482-489

[19] Liu J, Guaderrama N, Nager CW, Pretorius DH, Master S, Mittal RK. Functional correlates of anal canal anatomy: Puborectalis muscle and anal canal pressure. The American Journal of Gastroenterology. 2006;**101**(5):1092-1097

[20] Fox JC, Fletcher JG, Zinsmeister AR, et al. Effect of aging on anorectal and pelvic fl oor functions in females. Diseases of the Colon and Rectum. 2006;**49**(11):1726-1735

[21] Raza N, Bielefeldt K. Discriminative value of anorectal manometry in clinical practice. Digestive Diseases and Sciences. 2009;**54**(11):2503-2511

[22] Felt-Bersma RJ, Sloots CE, Poen AC, et al. Rectal compliance as a routine measurement: Extreme volumes have direct clinical impact and normal volumes exclude rectum as a problem. Diseases of the Colon and Rectum. 2000;**43**(12):1732-1738

[23] Ricciardi R, Mellgren AF, Madoff RD, et al. The utility of pudendal nerve terminal motor latencies in idiopathic incontinence. Diseases of the Colon and Rectum. 2006;**49**:852-857

[24] Pucciani F. Faecal soiling: Pathophysiology of postdefaecatory incontinence. Colorectal Disease. 2013;**15**:987-992

[25] Santoro GA, Wieczorek AP, Dietz HP, et al. State of the art: An integrated approach to pelvic floor ultrasonography. Ultrasound in Obstetrics and Gynecology. 2011;**37**:381-396

[26] Sudakoff GS, Quiroz F, Foley WD. Sonography of anorectal, rectal, and perirectal abnormalities. American Journal of Roentgenology. 2002;**179**:131-136

[27] Frudinger A, Bartram CI, Halligan S, et al. Examination techniques for endosonography of the anal canal. Abdominal Imaging. 1998;**23**(3):301

[28] Thakar R, Sultan AH. Anal endosonography and its role in assessing the incontinent patient. Best Practice and Research. Clinical Obstetrics and Gynaecology. 2004;**18**:157-173

[29] Abdool Z, Sultan AH, Thakar R. Ultrasound imaging of the anal sphincter complex: A review. The British Journal of Radiology. 2012;**85**:865-875

[30] Frudinger A, Halligan S, Bartram CI. Female anal sphincter: Age related differences in asymptomatic volunteers with high-frequency endoanal US. Radiology. 2002;**224**:417-423

[31] Mascagni D, Naldini G, Stuto A, et al. Recurrence after stapled haemorrhoidopexy. Techniques in Coloproctology. 2015;**19**:321-322

[32] Lengyel AJ, Hurst NG, Williams JG. Pre-operative assessment of anal fistulas using endoanal ultrasound. Colorectal Disease. 2002;**4**:436-440

[33] Pescatori M, Interisano A, Mascagni D, et al. Double flap technique to reconstruct the anal canal after concurrent surgery for fistulae, abscesses and haemorrhoids. International Journal of Colorectal Disease. 1995;**10**:19-21

[34] Navarro-Luna A, Garcia-Domingo MI, Rius-Macias JR, et al. Ultrasound study of anal fistulas with hydrogen peroxide enhancement. Diseases of the Colon and Rectum. 2004;**47**:108-114

[35] Ratto C, Gentile E, Merico M, et al. How can the assessment of fistula-in-ano be improved? Diseases of the Colon and Rectum. 2000;**43**:1375-1382

[36] Stoker J. Magnetic resonance imaging in fecal incontinence. Seminars in Ultrasound, CT, and MR. 2008;**29**:409-413

[37] Terra MP, Beets-Tan RG, van der, Hulst VPM, et al. MR imaging in evaluating atrophy of the external anal sphincter in patients with fecal incontinence. American Journal of Roentgenology. 2006;**187**(4):991-999

[38] Terra MP, Beets-Tan RG, van der Hulst VPM, et al. Anal sphincter defects in patients with fecal incontinence: Endoanal versus external phased-array MR imaging. Radiology. 2005;**236**:886-895

[39] Bharucha AE, Fletcher JG, Melton LJ III, Zinsmeister R. Obstetric trauma, pelvic floor injury and fecal incontinence: A population based case-control study. The American Journal of Gastroenterology. 2012;**107**:902-911

[40] Madoff RD. Surgical treatment options for fecal incontinence. Gastroenterology. 2004; **126**:S48-S54

[41] Schiedeck H, Schwandner O, Scheele J, Farke S, Bruch HP. Rectal prolapse: Which surgical option is appropriate? Langenbeck's Archives of Surgery. 2005;**390**:8-14

[42] Dobben AC, Terra MP, Slors JF, et al. External anal sphincter defects in patients with fecal incontinence: Comparison of endoanal MR imaging and endoanal US. Radiology. 2007;**242**:463-471

[43] Cazemier M, Terra MP, Stoker J, et al. Atrophy and defects detection of the external anal sphincter: Comparison between three-dimensional anal endosonography and endoanal magnetic resonance imaging. Diseases of the Colon and Rectum. 2005;**49**:20-27

[44] Dobben AC, Terra MP, Deutekom M, et al. The role of endoluminal imaging in clinical outcome of overlapping anterior anal sphincter repair in patients with fecal incontinence. American Journal of Roentgenology. 2007;**189**:W70-W77

[45] Malouf AJ, Halligan S, Williams AB, et al. Prospective assessment of interobserver agreement for endoanal MRI in fecal incontinence. Abdominal Imaging. 2001;**26**:76-78

[46] Townsend MK, Mattews CA, Whithehead WE, Grodstein F. Risk factors for fecal incontinence inolder women. The American Journal of Gastroenterology. 2013;**108**:113-119

[47] Umphred D. Neurological rehabilitation. St. Louis: MosbyElsevier; 2007

[48] Rao SSC. Current and emerging treatment options for fecal incontinence. Journal of Clinical Gastroenterology. 2014;**48**:752-764

[49] Scott KM. Pelvic floor rehabilitation in the treatment of fecal incontinence. Clinics in Colon and Rectal Surgery. 2014;**27**:99-105

[50] Meyer I, Richter HE. An evidence-based approach to the evaluation, diagnostic assessment and treatment of fecal incontinence in women. Current Obstetrics and Gynecology Reports. 2014;**3**:155-164

[51] van der Wilt AA, Giuliani G, Kubis C, van Wunnik BPW, Ferreira I, Breukink SO, Lehur PA, La Torre F, Baeten CGMI. Randomized clinical trial of percutaneous tibial nerve stimulation versus sham electrical stimulation in patients with faecal incontinence. The British Journal of Surgery. 2017 Aug;**104**(9):1167-1176

[52] Person B, Wexner SD. Advances in the surgical treatment of faecal incontinence. Surgical Innovation. 2005;**12**(1):7-21

[53] Barber MD, Bremer RE, Thor KB, Dolber PC, Kuehl TJ, Coates KW. Innervation of the female levator ani muscles. American Journal of Obstetrics and Gynecology. 2002;**187**(1): 64-71

[54] Grigorescu BA, Lazarou G, Olson T, Downie SA, Powers K, Greston WM, Mikhail MS. Innervation of the levator ani muscles: Description of the nerve branches to the pubococcygeus, iliococcygeus, and puborectalis muscles. International Urogynecology Journal. 2008;**19**:107-116

[55] Chan CLH, Ponsford S, Scott SM, Swash M, Lunniss PJ. Contribution of the pudendal nerve to sensation of the distal rectum. The British Journal of Surgery. 2005;**92**:859-865

[56] Matzel KE, Schmidt RA, Tanagho EA. Neuroanatomy of the striated muscular anal continence mechanism. Diseases of the Colon and Rectum. 1990;**33**(8):666-673

[57] Fowler CJ, Swinn MJ, Goodwin RJ, Oliver S, Craggs M. Studies of the latency of pelvic floor contraction during peripheral nerve evaluation show that the muscle response is refl exly mediated. The Journal of Urology. 2000;**163**(3):881

[58] Chancellor MB, Chartier-Kastler EJ. Principles of sacral nerve stimulation (SNS) for the treatment of bladder and urethral sphincter dysfunctions. Neuromodulation: Technology at the Neural Interface. 2000;**3**(1):16-26

[59] Blok BF, Groen J, Bosch JL, Veltman DJ, Lammertsma AA. Different brain effects during chronic and acute sacral neuromodulation in urge incontinent patients with implanted neurostimulators. BJU International. 2006;**98**:1238-1243

[60] Abdel-Halim MR, Crosbie J, Engledow A, Windsor A, Cohen CR, Emmanuel AV. Temporary sacral nerve stimulation alters rectal sensory function: A physiological study. Diseases of the Colon and Rectum. 2011;**54**:1134-1140

[61] Gourcerol G, Vitton V, Leroi AM, Michot F, Abysique A, Bouvier M. How sacral nerve stimulation works in patients with faecal incontinence. Colorectal Disease. 2011;**13**: e203-e211

[62] Watson NF. Anal bulking agents for faecal incontinence. Colorectal Disease. 2012 Dec; **14**(Suppl 3):29-33

[63] Guerra F, La Torre M, Giuliani G, Coletta D, Amore Bonapasta S, Velluti F, et al. Long-term evaluation of bulking agents for the treatment of fecal incontinence: Clinical outcomes and ultrasound evidence. Techniques in Coloproctology. 2015;**19**:23-27

[64] Hussain ZI, Lim M, Stojkovic SG. Systematic review of perianal implants in the treatment of fecal incontinence. The British Journal of Surgery. 2011;**98**:1526-1536

[65] Morris OJ, Smith S, Draganic B. Comparison of bulking agents in the treatment of faecal incontinence: A prospective randomized clinical trial. Techniques in Coloproctology. 2013;**17**:517-523

[66] La Torre F, de la Portilla F. Long-term efficacy of dex-tranomer in stabilized hyaluronic acid (NASHA/dx) for treatment of faecal incontinence. Colorectal Disease. 2013;**15**:569-574

[67] Ratto C, Parello A, Dionisi L, et al. Novel bulking agent for faecal incontinence. The British Journal of Surgery. 2011;**98**:1644-1652

[68] Ratto C, Buntzen S, Aigner F, Altomare DF, Heydari A, Donisi L, Lundby L, Parello A. Multicentre observational study of the gatekeeper for faecal incontinence. The British Journal of Surgery. 2016;**103**:290-299

[69] Al-Ozaibi L, Kazim Y, Hazim W, Al-Mazroui A, Al-Badri F. The gatekeeper™ for fecal incontinence: Another trial and error. International Journal of Surgery Case Reports. 2014;**5**:936-938

[70] de la Portilla F, Reyes-Díaz ML, Maestre MV, Jiménez-Rodríguez RM, García-Cabrera AM, Vázquez-Monchul JM, Díaz-Pavón JM, Padillo-Ruiz FC.Ultrasonographic evidence of Gatekeeper™ prosthesis migration in patients treated for faecal incontinence: A case series. International Journal of Colorectal Disease. 2017 Mar;**32**(3):437-440

[71] Christiansen J, Lorentzen M. Implantation of artificial sphincter for anal incontinence. Lancet. 1987;**2**:244e245

[72] Lehur PA, Michit F, Denis P, Grise P, Leborgne J, Teniere P, et al. Results of artificial sphincter in severe anal incontinence. Diseases of the Colon and Rectum. 1996;**39**:1352-1355

[73] Hong KD, Dasilva G, Kalaskar SN, et al. Long-term outcomes of artificial bowel sphincter for fecal incontinence: A systematic review and meta-analysis. Journal of the American College of Surgeons. 2013;**217**(4):718-725

[74] Wexner SD, Jin HY, Weiss EG, et al. Factors associated with failure of the artificial bowel sphincter: A study of over 50 cases from Cleveland Clinic Florida. Diseases of the Colon and Rectum. 2009;**52**:1550e1557

[75] Wong MT, Meurette G, Wyart V, et al. The artificial bowel sphincter: A single institution experience over a decade. Annals of Surgery. 2011;**254**(6):951

[76] Lee YY. What's new in the toolbox for constipation and fecal incontinence? Frontiers of Medicine (Lausanne). 2014;**1**:5

[77] Galandiuk S, Roth LA, Greene QJ. Anal incontinence sphincter ani repair: Indications, techniques, outcome. Langenbeck's Archives of Surgery. 2009;**394**(3):425-433

[78] Tan JJ, Chan M, Tjandra JJ. Evolving therapy for fecal incontinence. Diseases of the Colon and Rectum. 2007;**50**(11):1950-1967

[79] Edden Y, Wexner SD. Therapeutic devices for fecal incontinence: Dynamic graciloplasty, artificial bowel sphincter and sacral nerve stimulation. Expert Review of Medical Devices. 2009;**6**:307-312

[80] Person B, Wexner SD. Advances in the surgical treatment of fecal incontinence. Surgical Innovation. 2005;**12**(2):182

[81] Altomare DF, Dodi G, La Torre F, Romano G, Melega E, Rinaldi M. Multicentre retrospective analysis of the outcome of artificial anal sphincter implantation for severe faecal incontinence. The British Journal of Surgery. 2001;**88**(11):1481-1486

[82] La Torre F, Masoni L, Montori J, et al. The surgical treatment of fecal incontinence with artificial anal sphincter implant. Preliminary clinical report. Hepato-Gastroenterology. 2004;**51**:1358-1361

[83] Fernando RJ, Sultan AH, Kettle C, Thakar R. Methods of repair for obstetric anal sphincter injury. Cochrane Database of Systematic Reviews. 2013 Dec 8;**12**

[84] Premkumar G. Perineal trauma: Reducing associated postnatal maternal morbidity. RCM Midwives. 2005;**8**(1):30-32

[85] Fornell EU, Matthiesen L, Sjodahl R, Berg G. Obstetric anal sphincter injury ten years after: Subjective and objective long term effects. BJOG: An International Journal of Obstetrics and Gynaecology. 2005;**112**:312-316

[86] Rieger N, Wattchow D. The effect of vaginal delivery on anal function. The Australian and New Zealand Journal of Surgery. 1999;**69**:172-177

[87] Valsky DV, Lipschuetz M, Bord A, Eldar I, Messing B, Hochner-Celnikier D, Lavy Y, Cohen SM, Yagel S. Fetal head circumference and length of secondary stage ah labor are risk for levator ani muscle injury, diagnosed by 3-dimensional transperineal ultrasound in primiparous women. American Journal of Obstetrics and Gynecology. 2009;**201**:91-97

[88] Midwifery J, McCandlish R. Perineal trauma: Prevention and treatment. Women's Health. 2001;**46**(6):396-401

[89] Lamblin G, Bouvier P, Damon H, Chabert P, Moret S, Chene G, Mellier G. Long-term outcome after over lapping anterior anal sphincter repair for fecal incontinence. International Journal of Colorectal Disease. 2014;**29**:1377-1383

[90] Parks AG, McPartlin JF. Late repair of injuries of the anal sphincter. Proceedings of the Royal Society of Medicine. 1971;**64**(12):1187-1189

[91] Brown SR, Wadhawan H, Nelson RL. Surgery for faecal incontinence in adults. Cochrane Database of Systematic Reviews. 2013 Jul 2;**7**

[92] Walega P, Romaniszyn M, Siarkiewicz B, Zelazny D. Dynamic versus adynamic graciloplasty in treatmentof end-stage fecal incontinence: Is the implantation of the pacemaker really necessary? 12-month follow-up in a clinical, physiological, and functional study. Gastroenterology Research and Practice. 2015;**2015**:698516

[93] Vaizey CJ, Kamm MA, Nicholls RJ. Recent advances in the surgical treatment of faecal incontinence. The British Journal of Surgery. 1998;**85**:596-603

[94] Senapati A, Phillips RK. The trephine colostomy: A permanent left iliac fossa end colostomy without recourse to laparotomy. Annals of the Royal College of Surgeons of England. 1991;**73**:305-306

[95] Poirier M, Abcarian H. Fecal incontinence. In: Cameron JL, editor. Current Surgical Therapy. Philadelphia: Mosby Elsevier; 2008. pp. 285-291

Section 6

Hints of Colo-Rectal Surgery

Chapter 8

Clinical Pathway Evaluation for Left and Sigmoid Colectomy in Abdominal Surgery

Laurine Mattart, Marie Stevens, Nicolas Debergh, David Francart, Constant Jehaes, David Magis, Paul Magotteaux, Benoit Monami, Vanessa Verdin, Christian Wahlen, Joseph Weerts and Serge Markiewicz

Additional information is available at the end of the chapter

http://dx.doi.org/10.5772/intechopen.78588

Abstract

At the end of 2008, a new left colon clinical pathway was implemented in our hospital and set up by a multidisciplinary team, monitored by a clinical pathway coordinator. Our aim was to evaluate the quality of left and sigmoid colectomy management, to simplify the clinical pathway and to assess its impact on the patient, the medical and nursing staffs. A sample of 290 patients with benign or malignant disease requiring a laparoscopic of laparotomy left colon resection (mainly sigmoid) was included in this clinical pathway during the years 2009–2017. Our analysis focused particularly on the compliance with the protocol, the pain felt, the suture leak rate, the hospital stay, the re-hospitalization rate and redo surgery within 30 days. Our work leads to the conclusion that the introduction of a clinical pathway, when it is well prepared and brings together all the implicated persons with the same goal, is feasible with convincing results. These are directly beneficial to the patient and to the quality of its management.

Keywords: clinical pathway, left colon, laparoscopy, open colectomy, hospital stay, colon cancer

1. Introduction

A clinical pathway (CP) is an approach of multidisciplinary global management of a population with the same pathology or the same needs, aiming especially at the fast restitution of the physical and psychological capacities of the operated patient. It involves the establishment of a coordination between all the actors concerned by the therapeutic gesture and a specific organization of care, the patient playing an active role. The patient is no longer a sick, suffering person, he becomes an actor. For this active role to be effective, the patient must understand why he comes to the hospital, fully accept the medical procedures he will undergo and cooperate to return to the initial state as quickly as possible. With the information he receives, the patient must report on himself accurately and with the help of the medical and paramedical staff, define the physical and psychological situation at the best for him.

A CP brings coherence to the various therapeutic gestures from the preparation of the patient to his entry to the hospital until the end of his care, by the healthcare team after his return to home. The consistency in care, once perceived, is a reassuring factor for the patient who is facing a challenge. The CP will allow to sequence all the steps of the patient's journey and thus favor the optimization of the role of each of the actors in the care process. It is also a way to reassure the teams.

Clinical indicator
1. Managing the pain in pre, per, postoperative period (on a numerical scale, the pain should be ≤ 3 for the first 24 hours and ≤ 2 thereafter). Pain assessed at each break and documented in the medical record. During the peroperative period, patient controlled analgesia (PCA) is not planned for laparoscopy, but planned for laparotomy.
2. Follow-up of the resumption of the transit: recovery of the gases and stools indicated in the medical file (the patient is authorized to leave the hospital without saddles)
3. Follow-up of the food tolerance: nausea, vomiting filled in the medical file. Removing the gastric tube in the recovery room.
4. Follow-up of the temperature and keeping below 38°C
5. Follow-up of the wound: clean/dirty wound mentioned in the file
Department indicator
6. Patient information: distribution of a brochure during the preoperative consultation
Team indicator
7. Quality of the medical record, satisfaction of team work
Process indicator
8. Admission of the patient on day-1 if the surgery is scheduled before 10:00 am and on day 0 if it is scheduled after 10:00 am
9. For laparoscopy: removal of bladder catheter on day 1 or after day 1 with the reason indicated in the medical file. For laparotomy: removal on day 2 or after day 2 with the reason indicated in the medical file
10. Postoperative consultation four to six weeks after discharge of the patient of the hospital
11. Postoperative blood analysis on ≤ day 2
Financial indicator
12. Blood order without transfusion

Table 1. Clinical pathway protocol in the abdominal surgery department.

This chapter describes our first CP implemented in abdominal surgery in 2009 for the management of patients undergoing a colectomy. Such pathways of care in colorectal surgery were initiated in the 1990s [1] and are still the subject of numerous publications [2–4]. Left colon resections are performed in case of infection, tumor (benign or malignant) or inflammatory diseases. The objectives of such a resection are to remove the diseased colon, restore the digestive function closest to normal and avoid a colostomy. The feasibility of laparoscopic left colon resection for colon cancer, compared to laparotomy, was demonstrated [5]. Some complex conditions such as obesity, local tumor invasion or rectal tumor localization require in 5–15% of cases a conversion from laparoscopy to laparotomy.

With a follow-up of 9 years after the start of our CP, we analyzed the compliance of the actors to the CP protocol, the rate of suture leak, readmission or redo surgery. The CP is evaluated on the basis of a series of indicators involved in the three steps of the management of the operated patient: pre-, per- and postoperative periods.

The indicators selected concern the clinical state (the follow-up of the pain felt, resumption of transit, food tolerance, temperature, wound status), the service (patient information), the team (team work satisfaction), the process (patient admission, bladder catheter removal, postoperative consultation and blood analysis) and the financial aspects (order of blood bags without transfusion, number of complications) [6] (**Table 1**). Our objective is to study, on the basis of a wide range of data collected and analyzed painstakingly the impact of the implementation of a CP for left colectomy on all the nursing staff and the patient.

2. Patients and methods

2.1. Description of the population

Between January 01, 2009 and December 31, 2017, 265 consecutive patients with a median age of 64 (range 15–88) years old, with a male/female ratio of 1/0.9 and a median body mass index (BMI) of 25 kg/m^2 (range 16–40, obese with a BMI ≥ 30 kg/m^2 representing 16% of the population), were treated in our abdominal surgery department for a resection of the left colon by laparoscopy. On the same period of time, for the same indications and by the same team, 19 patients who had undergone laparotomy for colectomy and 6 patients whose laparoscopic surgery was converted to laparotomy were also included in the CP. There are many reasons for these conversions such as colic mobilization impossible, poor visibility, adiposity or colonoscopy leading to a significant air dilation of the colon. The median age of this group of 25 patients is 65 (range 34–88) years old, with a male/female ratio of 1/1.3 and a median BMI of 28 kg/m^2 (range 18–42, obese with a BMI ≥ 30 kg/m^2 representing 40% of the population).

These resections were performed for cancer or various benign pathologies (diverticular disease, Crohn's disease, benign polyp, volvulus) (**Figures 1** and **2**). Patients with type 1 diabetes, allergic to local anesthetics, epileptic or with intestinal obstruction were not included in the CP. Over this same period, 195 patients entered the CP and then were removed for various reasons: resection more extensive than expected, too many complications or on the basis of a medical decision.

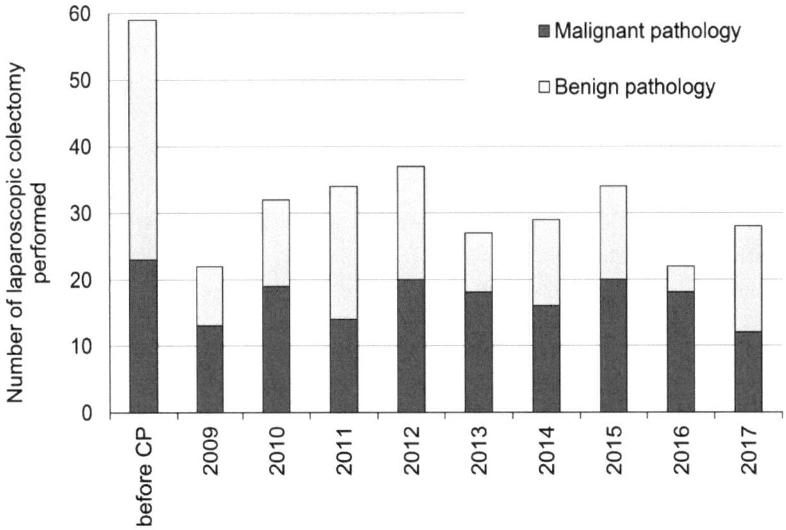

Figure 1. Number of laparoscopic surgery before (n = 59) and with the clinical pathway (CP) (n = 265).

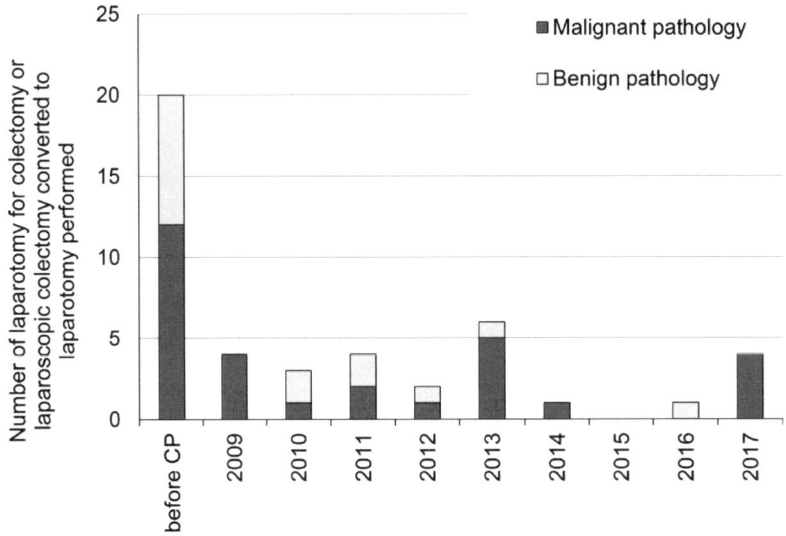

Figure 2. Number of laparotomy surgery before (n = 20) and with the clinical pathway (CP) (n = 25).

To evaluate the implementation of the CP, we compared the rate of suture leak, readmission and redo surgery and the length of stay to data obtained from consecutive series of patients who underwent resection of the left sigmoid colon between September 1, 2007 and August 31, 2008, with the same indications and by the same team but operated on in a conventional way. We chose a sufficiently recent period to avoid significant evolution in the healthcare, and sufficiently distant from the setting up of the CP to not be affected. Indeed, the therapeutic attitude of actors involved in the development of the CP protocol is inevitably affected by their readings and thoughts, before the implementation of the CP (see the section thereafter). This development period could encourage the emergence of new attitudes such as increased patient attention or systematic documentation of the medical record. For laparoscopies, we have a group of 59 patients with a median age of 60 (15–86) years old, with a male/female ratio of 1/0.7 and a median BMI of 25 kg/m^2 (19–38, obese with a BMI ≥ 30 kg/m^2 representing 14% of the population). We have a group of 14 laparotomies and 6 conversions with a median age of 75 (49–84) years old, with a male/female ratio of 1/1.2 and a median BMI of 28 kg/m^2 (15–38, obese with a BMI ≥ 30 kg/m^2 representing 27% of the population).

2.2. Implementation of the clinical pathway

The development of the CP, 1 year before its implementation, began with the establishment of a multidisciplinary CP project group that met monthly. This group is composed of two surgeons, two anesthesiologists, two nursing heads of surgical units, a nurse within the operating room, two social workers, two dieticians and the Liege Hospital Center nurse coordinator and project manager.

After evaluating the feasibility of the study, this group has: (1) developed the CP based on the analysis of the working method in the hospital and on best practices; (2) coordinated the daily working; (3) trained healthcare teams before and with the CP; (4) sensitized and followed the patients included; (5) performed the regular evaluation of the CP; and finally (6) continuously dispatched the results. The synthesis of the management consensus developed by the CP project group, and still applicable in 2018, is detailed (**Table 2**). This protocol is added to the basic protocol (cutaneous preparation, monitoring parameters, thromboprophylaxis, ...) of any patient operated on for abdominal surgery.

It seemed interesting to us to entrust the methodological aspect of the CP project to the CP nurse coordinator who is, by its specific function and motivation, the most available for the daily management of patient' needs and material constraints. This coordinator is required to have multiple contacts with each of the actors, doctors and paramedics. Placed at the center of the project, she will have a permanent overview of the CP and can propose any adjustments at any time to improve the consistency of the approach and its progression. After the establishment of the CP, the CP project group meets minimum once a year with the coordinator to examine what needs to be improved or modified. The whole CP was implemented "overnight" in each department concerned, within a single hospital.

2.3. Data management

To evaluate compliance, 12 parameters were analyzed as indicators: the time of admission of the patient, the pain assessment, the follow-up of the food tolerance, the follow-up of the temperature, the follow-up of the recovery of gases and stools, the follow-up of the wound condition, the time of the removal of the bladder catheter, the type of analgesic used, the order of blood without transfusion, the postoperative consultation and blood test. We define compliance as excellent when indicators are followed at least 80%. We carried out a simple evaluation to know if the protocol was respected, based on a YES/NO answer. When the goal is reached in consecutive years, the indicator is no longer evaluated and is noted NA for not assessed in **Table 3**.

Timing	
Day 1	Total body wash
Day 0 pre-operative	Carbohydrate loading (H-3) 2 fleet enema (H-2) Pre-operative sedation (H-1h30)
Day 0 per-operative	Intravenous fluid Antibiotic prophylaxis Preventive opioid sparing analgesic Normothermia Prevention of nausea and vomiting Lidocaine – ketamine IV TAP-block (laparotomy)
Day 0 post-operative	Avoidance of nasogastric tube TED prophylaxis Oral opioid sparing multimodal analgesia Early mobilisation out of bed Free liquids
Day 1	Free diet Early termination of IV fluid (laparoscopy) Early termination of uritary drainage (laparoscopy)
Day 2	Early termination of IV fluid (laparotomy) Early termination of uritary drainage (laparotomy)

Table 2. Clinical pathway for left colectomy.

The evaluation of the pain is carried out as of day 0 and until the discharge of the patient of the hospital, on a numerical scale of self-evaluation of 0–10 (0, no pain, 10, the maximum pain imaginable). Since the objective was to remain ≤3 for the first 24 h following the intervention, and ≤ 2 thereafter, a pain management protocol was developed by a multidisciplinary team and implemented in pre-, per- and postoperative. As the evaluation of pain has become systematic during the implementation of the CP, we have no point of comparison with patients in care before the CP.

Data are collected from paper and electronic medical records and analyzed with Microsoft Office Excel. The nonparametric Kruskal-Wallis test, performed with the statistical analysis software R was used to compare the length of stay between the "before CP" measurements and the measurements from 2009 to 2017 (all years combined), to compare the measures of all the years from 2009 to 2017 between them and to compare the length of stay between the two types of pathology—benign *versus* malignant—with each measure (before CP, 2009, 2010, 2011, 2012, 2013, 2014, 2015, 2016, 2017). A result is considered statistically significant if the P value is less than or equal to 0.05 and statistically highly significant if the P value is less than or equal to 0.001.

	2009	2010	2011	2012	2013	2014	2015	2016	2017	Total number of patients	Number of patients complying with the protocol
Clinical indicators											
Analgesia – PCA not planned	77%	44%	76%	70%	70%	80%	79%	82%	71%	265	190 (72 %)
Pain assessment	95%	97%	97%	97%	100%	90%	NA	NA	NA	182	175 (96 %)
Follow-up of the recovery of the gases	91%	75%	74%	62%	89%	93%	91%	82%	86%	265	216 (82 %)
Follow-up of the recovery of the stools	91%	91%	85%	70%	96%	97%	85%	86%	93%	265	232 (88 %)
Follow-up of the food tolerance	91%	100%	100%	100%	100%	100%	94%	82%	100%	265	257 (97 %)
Follow-up of the temperature	100%	97%	94%	95%	100%	100%	97%	91%	100%	265	257 (97 %)
Follow-up of the wound	75%	91%	94%	95%	100%	100%	85%	91%	NA	235	216 (92 %)
Process indicators											
Time of patient admission	53%	68%	100%	100%	100%	100%	100%	52%	96%	193	164 (85 %)
Time of removal of the bladder catheter	91%	81%	56%	65%	96%	79%	77%	61%	73%	254	190 (75 %)
Postoperative blood analysis	100%	97%	94%	92%	85%	93%	NA	NA	NA	182	170 (93 %)
Postoperative consultation	95%	91%	91%	95%	93%	NA	NA	NA	NA	152	141 (93 %)
Financial indicators											
Order of blood without transfusion	100%	100%	97%	100%	96%	100%	NA	NA	NA	182	180 (99 %)

Table 3. Compliance with the protocol of laparoscopic left colectomy.

3. Results

3.1. Protocol compliance

With the exception of the type of analgesic used, the time of removal of the bladder catheter and the time of patient admission, protocol compliance was excellent (> 80%) for laparoscopic patients (**Table 3**), for laparotomy or laparoscopy converted to laparotomy (**Table 4**). We have enough patients in the laparoscopy group to detail compliance by year. While this varies from year to year for analgesia, the time of removal of the bladder catheter and the time of admission of the patients, it remains >80% from the outset and at the same level throughout the period analyzed (**Table 3**).

	Total number of patients	Number of patients complying with the protocol
Clinical indicators		
Analgesia – PCA planned	25	18 (72 %)
Pain assessment	19	19 (100%)
Follow-up of the recovery of the gases	25	20 (80%)
Follow-up of the recovery of the stools	25	24 (96%)
Follow-up of the food tolerance	25	23 (92%)
Follow-up of the temperature	25	25 (100%)
Follow-up of the wound	21	17 (81%)
Process indicators		
Time of patient admission, laparotomy surgery	19	6 (32%)
Time of patient admission, laparoscopy converted in laparotomy	6	3 (50 %)
Time of removal of the bladder catheter	23	10 (43%)
Postoperative blood analysis	20	20 (100%)
Postoperative consultation	19	19 (100%)
Financial indicators		
Order of blood without transfusion	20	19 (95%)

Table 4. Compliance with the protocol of laparotomy left colectomy.

3.2. Pain assessment

Analysis of the data obtained revealed that, globally, laparoscopic surgery (**Figure 3**), laparotomy or laparoscopy converted to laparotomy (**Figure 4**) remains almost painless. Postoperative pain is slightly less after laparoscopy than after laparotomy for malignant diseases. The clinical relevance of the observed differences is a moot point given the low values (the median pain is 0, 1 or 2).

3.3. The outcome

The postoperative evolution and length of stay of patients managed with the CP protocol are compared to the results of the control group. The demographic characteristics of the two groups are similar. The implementation of the CP for patient operated by laparoscopy tend to improve the quality of care since we observe a decrease in the number of patients with suture leak, the main complication of this type of surgery, from 5/59 patients (8%) before the CP to 9/265 patients (3%) with the CP (**Table 5**). Before the CP (n = 59), we accounted for 3% of readmission and 3% of redo surgery. In IC (n = 265), 19 patients (7%) were readmitted to hospital, of which 6 patients (2%) underwent redo surgery within 30 days after the resection. Suture leak, abscess, pain and hematoma are the reasons of readmission after laparoscopic left colectomy. Finally, the positive consequence of setting up the CP is the reduction of the postoperative hospital stay. The statistical analysis of the results indicates that it was reduced in a highly significant manner ($P < 0.001$) as soon as the CP was introduced (**Figure 5**).

http://dx.doi.org/10.5772/intechopen.78588

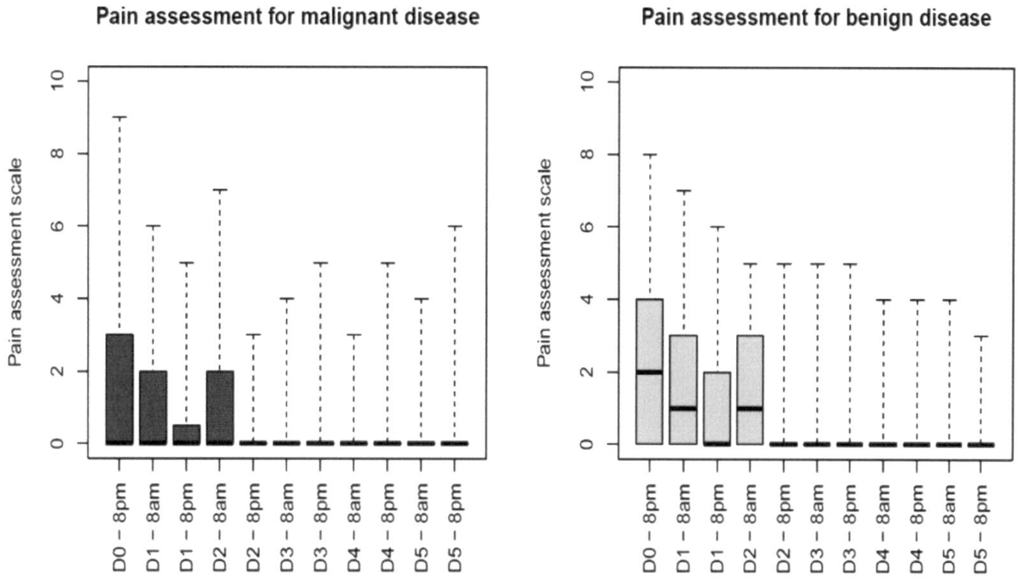

Figure 3. Pain assessment twice a day, patients operated by laparoscopy for malignant or benign pathology, included in the clinical pathway between 2009 and 2014 (n = 180). Minimum value – [lower quartile – median – upper quartile] – maximum value.

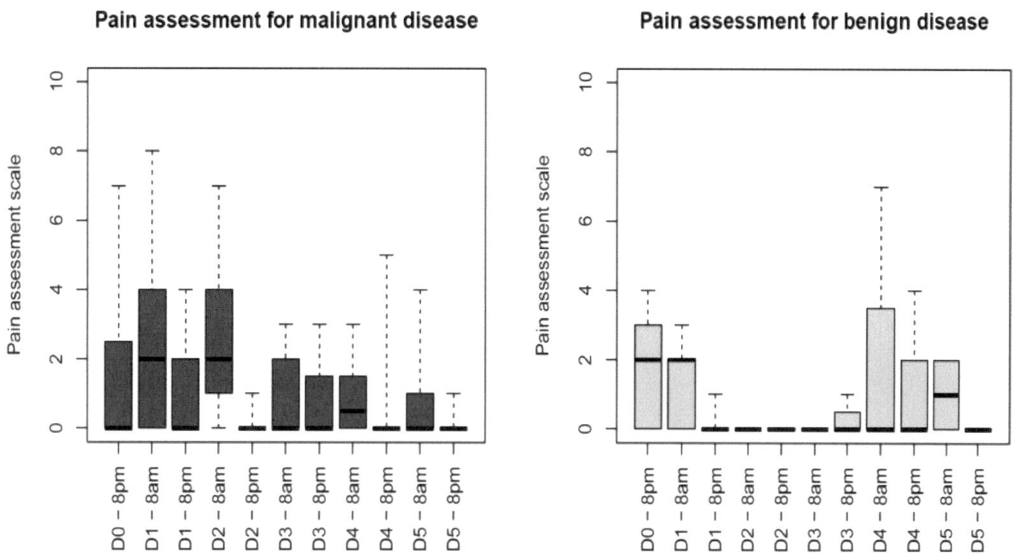

Figure 4. Pain assessment twice a day, patients operated by laparotomy for malignant or benign pathology, included in the clinical pathway between 2009 and 2014 (n = 19). Minimum value – [lower quartile – median – upper quartile] – maximum value.

The difference is observed between the measurements before CP and the measurement years 2009–2017 (all years combined). No difference was observed between the measurements from the years 2009–2017 (P = 0.853) and between the type of pathology, benign *versus* malignant, at

		Suture leak	Readmission	Redo surgery	Mean hospital stay (median, range)
Benign pathology	Before CP (n=36)	2 (6%)	2 (6%)	0%	5 days (6, 2-13)
	CP (n=115)	3 (3 %)	9 (8%)	1 (1 %)	4 days (4, 2-10)
Malignant pathology	Before CP (n=23)	3 (13%)	0%	2 (9%)	6 days (11, 3-45)
	CP (n=150)	6 (4 %)	10 (7 %)	5 (3 %)	4 days (4, 2-12)
Total	Before CP (n=59)	5 (8%)	2 (3%)	2 (3%)	5 days (8, 2-45)
	CP (n=265)	9 (3 %)	19 (7%)	6 (2 %)	4 days (4, 2-12)

Table 5. Mean hospital stay and complications within 30 days after laparoscopic left colectomy, patients managed before or during the clinical pathway (CP).

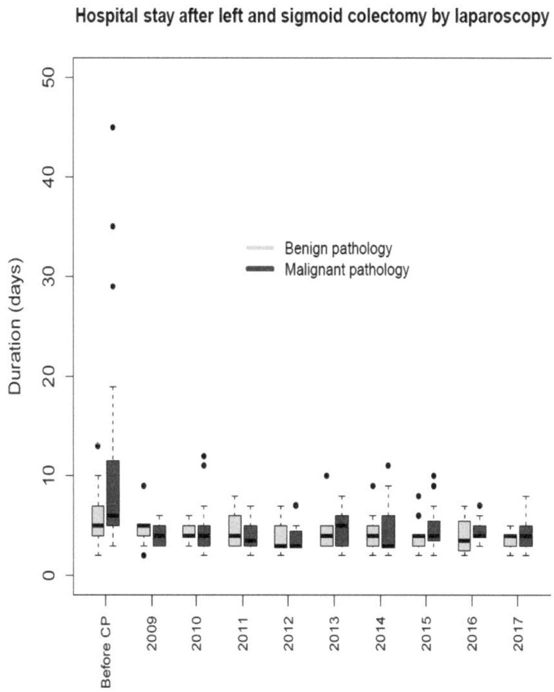

Figure 5. Box and whisker plot of the hospital stay after left (mainly sigmoid) colectomy by laparoscopy, for malignant (n = 150) or benign (n = 115) pathology, before or during the clinical pathway (CP). Minimum value – [lower quartile – median – upper quartile] –, maximum value. • outlier.

each measurement (P > 0.05). For malignant pathology, the median length of stay decreased by 7 days following the implementation of the CP, from 11 to 4 days (**Table 5**). For benign pathology, the median length of stay was 6 days before the CP and 4 days with the CP (**Table 5**).

		Suture leak	Readmission	Redo surgery	Mean hospital stay (median, range)
Benign pathology	Before CP (n=8)	0%	0%	0%	11 days (12, 4-23)
	CP (n=7)	0%	0%	0%	7 days (7, 4-13)
Malignant pathology	Before CP (n=12)	1 (8%)	1 (8%)	1 (8%)	10 days (11, 7-31)
	CP (n=18)	0%	1 (6%)	0%	7 days (7, 3-15)
Total	Before CP (n=20)	1 (5%)	1 (5%)	1 (5%)	10 days (12, 4-31)
	CP (n=25)	0%	1 (4%)	0%	7 days (7, 3-15)

Table 6. Mean hospital stay and complications within 30 days after laparotomy left colectomy, patients managed before or during the clinical pathway (CP).

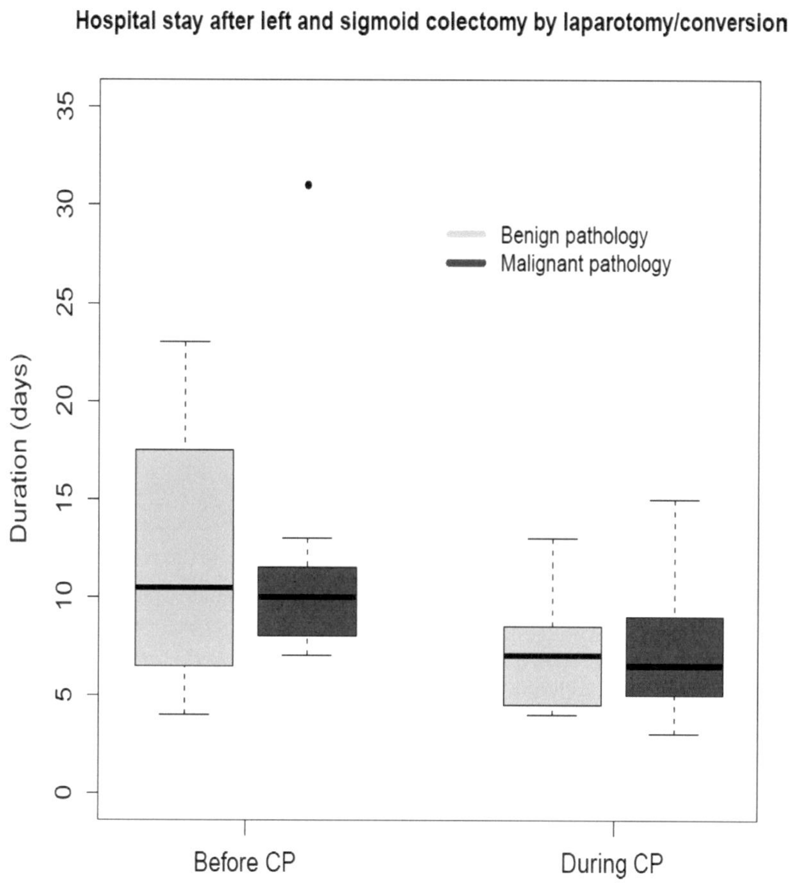

Figure 6. Box and whisker plot of the hospital stay after left (mainly sigmoid) colectomy by laparotomy, or by laparoscopy converted in laparotomy, for malignant (n = 18) or benign (n = 7) pathology, before or during the clinical pathway (CP). Minimum value – [lower quartile – median – upper quartile] – maximum value • outlier.

After the analysis of the group of 25 patients who underwent laparotomy for colectomy or complicated laparoscopic colectomy that required conversion to laparotomy, we note that the implementation of the CP did not affect the rates of suture leak, readmission or redo surgery within 30 days after the surgery. These rates were low before the CP (5% for each of the three studied parameters) and remained between 0 and 4% (**Table 6**). Flow of the lower part of the scar and fall with fracture of the right tibia are the reasons of readmission after laparotomy left colectomy. When we compare the length of hospital stay for this type of surgery before and with the CP, benign and malignant pathologies combined, we find that it decreased significantly ($P < 0.01$) with a median of 12 days of hospitalization before CP and 7 days with the CP (**Table 6** and **Figure 6**). No significant difference was observed between benign and malignant pathologies before the introduction of the CP ($P = 0.786$) or with the CP ($P = 1.000$). There are too few data per year to make effective comparisons.

No patients died within 30 days after the colectomy for the whole population including both control group ($n = 63$) and group in the CP ($n = 290$).

4. Discussion

This chapter describes the creation and implementation of a new protocol for colectomy of the left colon, mainly sigmoid, by abdominal surgeons at the Liege Hospital Center to improve the quality of care, the efficiency of health services and to reduce the variability of unjustified practices. This CP provides a healthcare pathway for laparoscopies, laparotomies and conversions from laparoscopy to laparotomy, supported for the same type of pathology, by the same team. A total of 290 resections were performed with the CP during 9 years, 265 laparoscopies procedures, 6 laparoscopies that required conversion to laparotomy and 19 laparotomies. This 2% of conversion rate is low compared to that described in the literature which is 5–15% [7, 8].

Through the precise codification of therapeutic gestures (**Table 1**), patient care and multidisciplinary teamwork have been improved. Medical, nursing and paramedical personnel appreciated the standardization of procedures, precise instructions, improvement of the quality of the patient's file, enhancement of multidisciplinary respect and collaboration. Although the recommendations show that a CP has a beneficial effect on patient management, its implementation in daily practice and its maintenance over time encounter certain difficulties due to the problems of effective coordination of the actors or the individualism of some. Procedures related to the organization of healthcare can cause significant resistance due to the impression that a margin of autonomy is being removed. The implementation of an IC also requires a change of mentality at the level of the patient, the medical and nursing staff, a modification of the habits rooted solidly in the practice of the various traditions, often based on nonupdated knowledge. Thus, although the protocol provides for the admission of patients on the day of the surgery if it is scheduled after 10:00 am, 68% of the patients operated on by laparotomy were admitted to the hospital the day before the surgical intervention even if it is scheduled after 10:00 am (**Table 4**). This additional time in the hospital before surgery could help to prepare him carefully to what awaits him, review with him the goal to achieve, avoid or reduce anxiety and emotional stress. Some patients would also be admitted sooner if the bowel preparation is too long.

It should be noted that the CP is not against the therapeutic freedom: it is an ideal pathway, not an obligation and always adapted to the patient. In this regard, a low compliance with the protocol is noted for the time of removal of the bladder catheter. For fear of having to re-catheterize the patient, the removal of the catheter was delayed on day 2 (instead of day 1 planned by the CP protocol) for 57% of the patient operated by laparoscopic surgery and on day 4 (instead of day 2) for 25% of patients operated by laparotomy/conversion. Although the presence of the tubes hampers the mobilization and the autonomy of the patient, this conscious transgression of the CP protocol aims for the well-being of the patient. It is the same for analgesia. Based on a medical decision, a patient controlled analgesia (PCA) was put for 28% of the patients operated by laparoscopy (**Table 3**), whereas the protocol does not predict it, and on the contrary, a PCA was not used for 28% of the patients operated by laparotomy (**Table 4**), whereas PCA is provided by the CP protocol.

For the majority of the criteria analyzed, compliance is not always excellent, varies from one year to another, or gradually improves (**Table 3**). This is explained by the fact that the medical and nursing staff does not always have the reflex to document the care in the medical file or has simply given up the follow-up of the CP protocol. Compliance with the CP protocol is also based on the excellent collaboration that existed within the department of abdominal surgery between doctors and healthcare staff before the implementation of this one. Establishing a collaboration between teams is like putting oil in the wheels. To implement a CP is to improve the quality of the oil already present in the wheels. Finally, the compliance to the protocol the "left colectomy CP" is also explained by the fact that it enjoys support from the management of the hospital, with the benefits that this implies, as explained by a team from Milan [9]. At Liege Hospital Center, CP are part of the " AZIMUT " strategic plan, in the " patient orientation and clinical efficiency " axis, which aims to redefine the configuration of the network and the offer of care offered to patients. Although complex, the study of the compliance with the CP protocol is an important point for us, which gives us information on the level of agreement between the recommendations of the CP and the practice, on the effectiveness of the CP. It is rarely presented in studies assessing the impact of a CP implementation [10].

By rethinking the management of patients and introducing a CP specific to laparoscopic left colectomy, we have shown that the quality of care is increased, without affecting the rate of complications which remains low compared to those published in the literature [4, 8, 11–14], and the hospital stay is significantly reduced (**Tables 5** and **6**). A limitation of our study is that the comparison group is a historical group and not a synchronous group, which should encourage caution in the final conclusions. Nevertheless, similar results have been published regarding laparoscopic colorectal surgery [4]. Various studies of laparoscopic left colon resection for diverticular disease described a median hospital stay of 7 days, with 4% of redo surgery (8 patients/205) [11], or an average hospital stay of 9 days, with 3% of suture leak and 2% of redo surgery [12]. For the malignant pathology, a mean hospital stay of 8 days [13] or a median hospital stay of 5 days with 12% of readmission and less than 2% of redo surgery were described [14]. Finally, for both types of pathology after left colectomy by laparoscopic surgery, we observe an average length of stay of 4 days, 7% of readmission and 2% of redo surgery, compared to 6 days, 6% of readmission and 6% of redo surgery in the literature [8]. Following a laparotomy or a laparoscopy converted in laparotomy, we observe an average length of stay of 7 days. This is comparable or even shorter than the results presented in the literature [7, 13]. Note that hospitalization is longer after laparotomy than laparoscopy (**Tables 5** and **6**). This may be related to ileus, possible postoperative pain and less significant overall morbidity for patients operated by laparoscopy [7, 15].

This new CP was developed and implemented by this multidisciplinary team and monitored by the CP coordinator. This would be the best "cocktail" to change perioperative habits [16]. The CP coordinator ensures that the program runs smoothly, with optimal patient supervision, especially during the preoperative period. The CP coordinator organizes a continuous evaluation of the CP and the results are systematically communicated to the different people involved. This regular and effective evaluation of care practices is essential because doctors and paramedics change, old habits identified as penalizing the CP come back easily, advances in medicine must be taken into account. If the value of the CP relies on the different actors and on the quality of the established protocol, it is clear that the expected success depends largely on the compliance of the patients to this kind of care. This involves focusing of the efforts of the healthcare team on the patient preparation and conditioning. He must sense that he is the main actor of the success of his therapy. In concrete terms, the patient receives a personalized message, a roadmap where the procedure is explained. He must be able to ensure his course. As soon as he gets back to his room after the surgery, he knows what to eat and how much to avoid nausea, if he wishes he can drink water, sit on the edge of the bed, on a chair or do few steps. In addition, we care in a continuous process of improvement based on patient feedback and assessments.

Our study shows that it is possible to implement a CP in a surgical department with convincing results as soon as it is put in place. This work was made possible only after a careful study of the different steps of the CP from the reception of the patient to the hospital, through the anesthesia and surgery department, the social worker, the general practitioner, the home care nurse and after having adapted all the logistic, psychological and economic factors to the reality of the field to finally obtain a process of original care, which meets the unanimity of the actors. Asking the purpose of the CP is frequent. One should not give the impression that it is imposed to the team. Moreover, the CP was set up overnight. This particularity was made possible thanks to the positive dynamics and devotion of the care providers and patients, thanks to a long, precise and complete preparation so that each actor knew precisely the role he had to assume and knowing his position in all steps listed in the CP. Previous studies have shown that the implementation time of such a program often takes much longer [16, 17].

5. Conclusion

Implemented in 2009, this CP brings coherence to all the management of left colon resection. The essential points of the CP are a good information to the patient who is the driving force of the process, a CP protocol meticulously created by all the actors and validated in multidisciplinary way, a regular follow-up by the CP coordinator and … the abandonment of a series of dogmas that turns out useless. Compliance with the project was remarkably high as soon as it started and remained constant for the next 9 years. The data systematically recorded shows that CP improves quality of care, promotes patient involvement, coordination and multidisciplinary collaboration. In addition, without increasing the number of complications and taking into account the risks associated with this type of surgery, there is a significant reduction in the length of stay. This analysis is part of the quality control at the base of any improvement in the overall care of patients. Each actors, patient and caregiver, have the will to make quality and to keep improving it.

Abbreviations

PCA	patient controlled analgesia
CP	clinical pathway
BMI	body mass index

Author details

Laurine Mattart[1]*, Marie Stevens[2], Nicolas Debergh[4], David Francart[4], Constant Jehaes[4], David Magis[3], Paul Magotteaux[1], Benoit Monami[4], Vanessa Verdin[4], Christian Wahlen[4], Joseph Weerts[4] and Serge Markiewicz[4]

*Address all correspondence to: laurine.mattart@chc.be

1 Quality Control Unit, Department of Abdominal Surgery, CHC Liege Hospital Center, Belgium

2 Clinical Pathway Unit, CHC Liege Hospital Center, Belgium

3 Department of Education, University of Liege, Belgium

4 Department of Abdominal Surgery, CHC Liege Hospital Center, Belgium

References

[1] Kehlet. Multimodal approach to control postoperative pathophysiology and rehabilitation. British Journal of Anaesthesia. 1997 May;**78**(5):606-617. PMID: 9175983

[2] Greco M, Capretti G, Beretta L, Gemma M, Pecorelli N, Braga M. Enhanced recovery program in colorectal surgery: A meta-analysis of randomized controlled trials. World Journal of Surgery. 2014 Jun;**38**(6):1531-1541. DOI: 10.1007/s00268-013-2416-8

[3] ERAS compliance group. The impact of enhanced recovery protocol compliance on elective colorectal cancer resection: Results from an international registry. Annals of Surgery. 2015 Jun;**261**(6):1153-1159. DOI: 10.1097/SLA.0000000000001029

[4] McEvoy MD, Wanderer JP, King AB, Geiger TM, Tiwari V, Terekhov M, Ehrenfeld JM, Furman WR, Lee LA, Sandberg WS. A perioperative consult service results in reduction in cost and length of stay for colorectal surgical patients: Evidence from a healthcare redesign project. Perioperative Medicine (London, England). 2016 Feb 5;**5**(3). DOI: 10.1186/s13741-016-0028-1

[5] Reza MM, Blasco JA, Andradas E, Cantero R, Mayol J. Systematic review of laparoscopic versus open surgery for colorectal cancer. The British Journal of Surgery. 2006 Aug;**93**(8):921-928. DOI: 10.1002/bjs.5430

[6] Vanhaecht K. The impact of clinical pathways on the organisation of care processes [thesis]. Katholieke Universiteit Leuven; ISBN-Number: 9789081222211; 2007

[7] Braga M, Vignali A, Gianotti L, Zuliani W, Radaelli G, Gruarin P, Dellabona P, Di Carlo V. Laparoscopic versus open colorectal surgery. A randomized trial on short-term outcome. Annals of Surgery. 2002 Dec;**236**(6):759-766. Discussion 767. DOI: 10.1097/01.SLA.0000036269.60340.AE

[8] Maitra RK, Acheson AG, Gornall C, Scholefield JH, Williams JP, Maxwell-Armstrong CA. Results of laparoscopic colorectal surgery from a national training center. Asian Journal of Surgery. 2014 Jan;**37**(1):1-7. DOI: 10.1016/j.asjsur.2013.07.005

[9] Bona S, Molteni M, Rosati R, Elmore U, Bagnoli P, Monzani R, Caravaca M, Montorsi M. Introducing an enhanced recovery after surgery program in colorectal surgery: A single center experience. World Journal of Gastroenterology. 2014 Dec 14;**20**(46):17578-17587. DOI: 10.3748/wjg.v20.i46.17578

[10] van Zelm R, Janssen I, Vanhaecht K, de Buck van Overstraeten A, Panella M, Sermeus W, Coeckelberghs E. Development of a model care pathway for adults undergoing colorectal cancer surgery: Evidence-based key interventions and indicators. Journal of Evaluation in Clinical Practice. 2018 Feb;**24**(1):232-239. DOI: 10.1111/jep.12700

[11] Pinto JO, Fallatah B, Espalieu P, Poncet G, Bissery A, Pinheiro FAS, Boulez JC. Elective laparoscopic left colectomy for diverticular disease: A monocentric study on 205 consecutive patients [Internet]. Arquivos Brasileiros de Cirurgia Digestiva. 2010;**23**(4):234-239. DOI: 10.1590/S0102-67202010000400005. [Accessed: March 01, 2018]

[12] Trebuchet G, Lechaux D, Lecalve JL. Laparoscopic left colon resection for diverticular disease. Surgical Endoscopy. 2002 Jan;**16**(1):18-21. DOI: 10.1007/s004640090122

[13] Desiderio J, Trastulli S, Ricci F, Penzo J, Cirocchi R, Farinacci F, Boselli C, Noya G, Redler A, Santoro A, Parisi A. Laparoscopic versus open left colectomy in patients with sigmoid colon cancer: Prospective cohort study with long-term follow-up. International Journal of Surgery. 2014;**12**(8):745-750. DOI: 10.1016/j.ijsu.2014.05.074

[14] Clinical Outcomes of Surgical Therapy Study Group, Nelson H, Sargent DJ, Wieand HS, Fleshman J, Anvari M, Stryker SJ, Beart RW Jr, Hellinger M, Flanagan R Jr, Peters W, Ota D. A comparison of laparoscopically assisted and open colectomy for colon cancer. The New England Journal of Medicine. 2004 May 13;**350**(20):2050-2059. DOI: 10.1056/NEJMoa032651

[15] King PM, Blazeby JM, Ewings P, Franks PJ, Longman RJ, Kendrick AH, Kipling RM, Kennedy RH. Randomized clinical trial comparing laparoscopic and open surgery for colorectal cancer within an enhanced recovery programme. The British Journal of Surgery. 2006 Mar;**93**(3):300-308. DOI: 10.1002/bjs.5216

[16] Pędziwiatr M, Kisialeuski M, Wierdak M, Stanek M, Natkaniec M, Matłok M, Major P, Małczak P, Budzyński A. Early implementation of enhanced recovery after surgery (ERAS) protocol – Compliance improves outcomes: A prospective cohort study. International Journal of Surgery. 2015 Sep;**21**:75-81. DOI: 10.1016/j.ijsu.2015.06.087

[17] Ahmed J, Khan S, Lim M, Chandrasekaran TV, MacFie J. Enhanced recovery after surgery protocols - compliance and variations in practice during routine colorectal surgery. Colorectal Disease. 2012 Sep;**14**(9):1045-1051. DOI: 10.1111/j.1463-1318.2011.02856.x